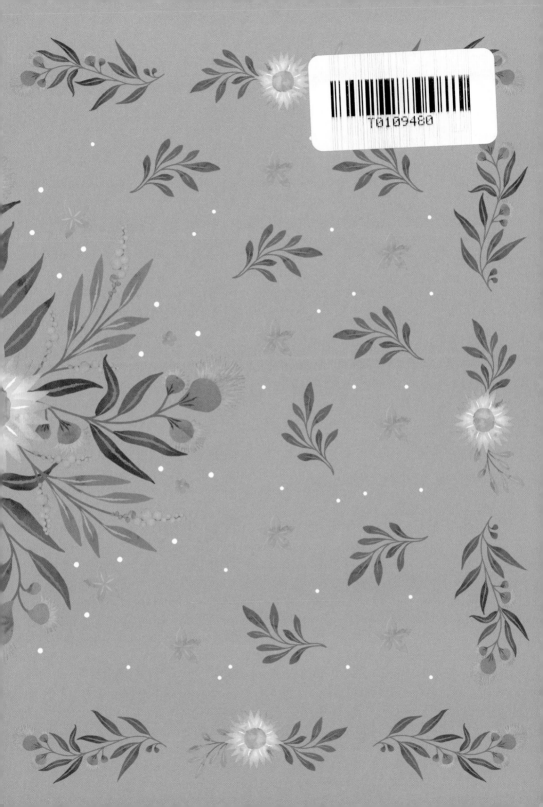

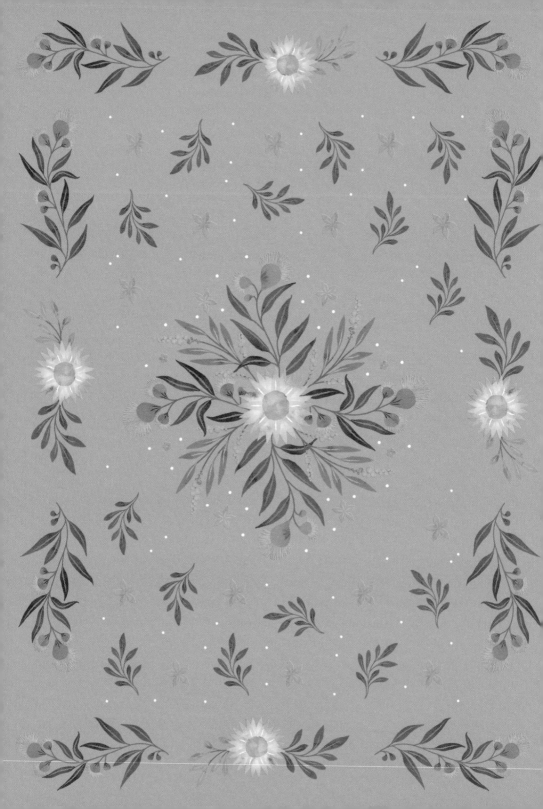

My Wellness
JOURNAL

Connect to your body
Balance your hormones
Improve your health

Melissa Christie and
Stephanie Crane

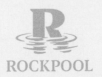

ROCKPOOL

About the creators

Melissa Christie is an author, speaker, co-host of *The PCOS Girls Podcast*, PCOS fertility coach and mum to two rainbow babies. After a diagnosis with PCOS and the miscarriage of her first baby, Melissa began a healing journey that revealed to her just how segmented the health industry was. Melissa began sharing her belief that to heal and maintain health, we need to understand our own body and advocate for it and become aware of the many approaches we can take to healing, including those outside of western medicine. She released her first book and began receiving messages of pregnancies and improved symptoms because of the information she had shared. She became a fluent speaker on periods, hormones and fertility and an advocate for getting information about these topics taught in schools. Melissa currently spends her days running her business, growing with her family and slipping in self-care practices every chance she gets.

Stephanie Crane is a graphic designer and henna artist with a passion for meaningful projects. Along with her passion for the bush and for fighting fires, she has found her purpose in art. Stephanie spends her days with her family, working by the fire with her baby, in the little cottage she built.

Who is this journal for?

This journal is for people of any gender who are on a journey with periods, pregnancy or perimenopause, and the symptoms and conditions that can affect those phases of life.

In saying that, the hormonal profiles, journeys, challenges and experiences on the gender spectrum are diverse, and one journal cannot encapsulate it all or suit everybody. As cis-women creating this journal from a patient-perspective, we don't have the lived experience or expert knowledge to properly convey the nuances of health care and health advocacy needed for a well-rounded journal for people on a journey with gender affirming hormonal therapy. But we do hope to one day see a journal like that on the shelf.

In this journal, we do occasionally use the terms 'women', 'girls' and 'female' when quoting relevant research and statistics that reference these terms themselves. We are reporting these findings as they are written, because reporting it any other way would possibly be misleading of the researchers' intentions and the outcomes of the research. But we want to acknowledge that when we do this, we are not conveying our personal assumption of the gender of the participants or the misconception that the research is only relevant to women.

It is so important to us that this journal is inclusive. Of course, we wouldn't want to offend or harm anyone. But ultimately, we have written this journal inclusively because it is the most accurate thing to do – the symptoms, conditions and experiences explored throughout this journal simply do not exclusively affect people who identify as women, and we want this information to help protect and improve the health of all who are on this journey with us.

How to use your journal

This journal is undated, meaning you can start it on any day of any year. It's divided into two sections and you will use both sections daily. The first section contains 52 weeks of journal space. This is where you record and reflect on the day-to-day stuff, like how much sleep you're getting, your meals and your water intake.

The first section is also broken into chapters. Each chapter will help you knowledge-up on factual, practical info about how the body works, the health conditions that can affect us, and the multitude of ways we can protect and improve our health. You will learn something new every week and at the end of each chapter, you will have an opportunity to reflect on the knowledge you've gained.

The second section contains 12 months of charts. This is where you track and monitor the big stuff, like your cycle, symptoms, test results and treatments.

We suggest you work through the journal from beginning to end, but if there's a chapter you'd rather tackle first, go for it – the journal works wherever you start.

At the very back of the journal, you will find a section to reflect on the year that was and some general notes pages where you can write down things you learn that you don't want to forget or things you would like to bring up with your doctor.

Before all that though, to get you up to speed on some of the basics, convey what this journal is all about and get you kickstarted on your journey, take a bit of time to absorb the next few pages . . .

CONTENTS

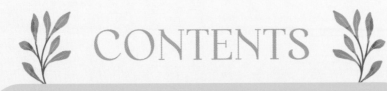

INTRODUCTION   1

Welcome to your journal . . .   1

Your weekly journal space   3

Intentions for the year   4

WEEKLY JOURNAL SECTION   5

Chapter 1: Let's get those basics   5

Chapter 2: Can we get a little support up in here?   29

Chapter 3: Periods and hormones and cycles – oh my!   51

Chapter 4: Fertility (psst . . . even if you never want to have
a baby – don't skip this section! Your fertility
still matters!)   81

Chapter 5: Mental health . . . AKA health   107

Chapter 6: The gut – who even knew it was the epicentre
of health?   137

Chapter 7: Hello thyroid   155

Chapter 8: When it comes to nutrition – you do you   173

Chapter 9: Self-care practices that actually heal   203

MONTHLY CHARTS   233

LET'S REFLECT   310

Welcome to your journal

F riend! How good are you?! Having this journal is a total, tangible commitment to your health and that's a big deal. To ensure the weight of this moment isn't wasted, we've decided to start by getting pretty real.

And by real, we mean slightly heavy – but necessary.

So grab your beverage of choice and settle in . . .

The truth is – this journal shouldn't need to exist.

The information contained in these pages *should* be taught in school as a matter of priority. It should be taught so thoroughly that it is engrained knowledge – like knowing that the sun keeps us warm and that grass needs water to grow.

The fact that it isn't taught to us in this way is a disservice and it's affecting our health. Research has found that body literacy – AKA the understanding of how the body works and how health practices and conditions affect *your* body – is essential for people's health. We *need* to understand health to improve our chances of remaining healthy.

So *My Wellness Journal* is here. It's here to impart everything you have a right to know about cycles and fertility and how all the systems of our body are connected in this incredible, genuinely mind-blowing way.

From this journal you can expect to gain a deep understanding of how our nutrition and lifestyle can affect our body, how we can use the phases of our cycle to our advantage, the many natural medicines that can help us, the conditions that can affect us, the tips and tricks that can add to your wisdom as a person in your community, and the serious importance and power of dedicating time to self-care.

Importantly, you will also gain a thorough understanding of *your* body, a resolute passion for prioritising your health and a framework to help you understand how to advocate for your health.

Because currently, health *is* a matter of advocacy. The context in which we receive health care is a feminist issue of informed consent and medical gaslighting, and some medical practices and treatments that were created decades ago are failing us. And so many of us are suffering needlessly because of it.

As you read this journal, you may come to decide that it's time to demand change so we can live in a world where body literacy is fostered from childhood, we are engrained with a positive relationship with our body and cycle, and the health system supports us *with* informed consent and *without* bias.

The information in this journal is told to you in an open, do-with-it-what-you-will kind of way. This journal does not exist to push a singular approach upon you or judge the choices you make. We are all different. Different foods and medicines work in different ways for different bodies. In this journal, we share a wide range of approaches to health across multiple modalities – from functional medicine to naturopathy to Chinese medicine, so your knowledge can grow and you can find a path that leads you on a journey that suits *you*.

This journey starts with you and it begins on the very next page of this journal. We swear it's more fun than this weighty introduction.

In happiness and health,

Mel and Steph

@pcospathways | @sleepyhollowcreative

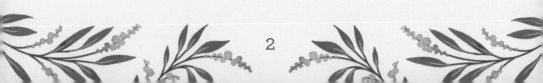

Your weekly journal space

This section is organised by weeks and is divided into chapters. Each week contains space for you to plan your meals and track your body movement, sleep, self-care, water intake and gratitude. It also has prompts to motivate and inspire you and to help you reflect on the week that was.

Spread throughout this section is tonnes of info about health. Each week, you will deep dive on a topic (or two) and be given plenty of tips that are bite-sized and easy to read.

And don't forget to check out the monthly charts section at the back of the journal, to track all the big things, like your cycle, symptoms, test results and treatments. And if you don't know how to track your cycle, don't worry. Over the next couple of weeks, you're going to learn all about it.

Intentions for the year

This page is a space for you to sink into how you want to approach the year. Your intentions or goals can be powerful motivators and can provide some really supportive direction.

For those of you who are goal oriented, this is a great place for writing your goals and thinking about the steps you could take to achieve them.

For those of you who don't like setting goals, you can use this space to record your intentions or inspiring thoughts for the year.

_____

_____

_____

_____

_____

_____

_____

_____

_____

_____

_____

_____

_____

_____

_____

_____

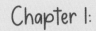

LET'S GET THOSE BASICS

hen it comes to health, there's a lot that gets missed when we're at school. And even more that gets brushed over in society. This chapter is all about ensuring you've got the fundamentals under wraps.

By the end of this chapter, you will understand all you need to know about ovulation and tracking your cycle, what your reproductive system looks like and some essential knowledge about hormone health.

You will hopefully also feel a lot more comfortable with the idea of sharing what you know and talking about your experiences.

What is ovulation and how does it occur?

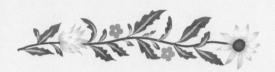

If you want to understand, support and improve your health, then no matter your goals, understanding ovulation and how it works is important. Ovulation is a reflection of our health and being aware of it can add depth to the understanding of how your body works.

WHAT EXACTLY IS OVULATION?

Ovulation is an event that happens during our cycle, where an egg is released from one of our ovaries.

Ovaries contain fluid-filled sacs called follicles that each contain eggs. We have two ovaries and, typically, the one releasing the egg alternates each cycle.

Once the egg is released, it is either fertilised by sperm and becomes an embryo, or it is released from your body during your period.

Sounds simple enough, but there is an amazingly intricate stream of events that needs to occur within your body for ovulation to happen.

HOW DOES IT HAPPEN?

To ovulate, the body releases a range of hormones at specific times. Hormones are like messages that tell cells in certain parts of your body what to do.

There are organs in our body that produce our hormones. The HPO axis consists of three of these organs — the hypothalamus and pituitary gland (both located in the brain) and the ovaries, which are located in our pelvis. The HPO axis is what produces the hormones we need to ovulate.

While hormonal imbalances (like in someone with polycystic ovary syndrome, or PCOS) can throw all of this out of whack, here is how a typical cycle unfolds:

- From the first day of our period, our body is in the follicular phase and our hypothalamus releases gonadotrophin-releasing hormone (GnRH) and our pituitary gland produces follicle-stimulating hormone (FSH) and luteinising hormone (LH).

- FSH tells our ovaries to prepare one egg for ovulation. It also stimulates the follicles to make estradiol, our main estrogen. Estradiol thickens the uterine lining (in case you become pregnant and an embryo needs to embed in the lining) but it's also beneficial for general health.

- The follicle that is largest will become the dominant follicle, which will end up releasing its egg.

- Estrogen levels peak as the follicle grows to about 2 cm to 3 cm and sends a signal to the pituitary gland to release a surge of LH.

- The LH surge triggers the follicle to release its egg into the fallopian tube – this is ovulation and it typically occurs around day 14 of your cycle, but anytime between day 7 and day 28 can be normal.

- Your body is now in its luteal phase and that dominant follicle turns into your corpus luteum (a fully fledged organ that your body creates and destroys every cycle).

- Your corpus luteum produces progesterone and estrogen to support your egg if it becomes fertilised. Progesterone also provides beneficial feedback to the hypothalamus to slow the release of LH and therefore prevent androgen excess (more on that later).

- If your egg is fertilised, it will embed in your uterine lining and the corpus luteum will continue to produce progesterone to support early pregnancy (it will break down at about 12 weeks' gestation when the baby takes over the production of progesterone).

- If your egg isn't fertilised, your corpus luteum will start to break down about 10 days after you ovulate, lowering progesterone and estrogen levels, causing you to get your period.

- It is also possible to get your period *without* having ovulated. That is an anovulatory cycle, which is common with PCOS.

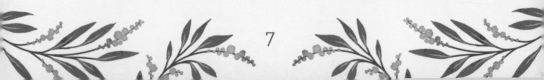

WEEK 1

Intention for the week:

MONDAY

SELF-CARE	MEAL PLAN	BODY MOVEMENT
Zz		

Today I am grateful for:

TUESDAY

SELF-CARE	MEAL PLAN	BODY MOVEMENT
Zz		

Today I am grateful for:

WEDNESDAY

SELF-CARE	MEAL PLAN	BODY MOVEMENT
Zz		

Today I am grateful for:

THURSDAY

SELF-CARE	MEAL PLAN	BODY MOVEMENT
Zz		

Today I am grateful for:

'No one saves us but ourselves. No one can and no one may. We ourselves must walk the path.' – BUDDHA

FRIDAY

SELF-CARE	MEAL PLAN	BODY MOVEMENT

Z^zz

Today I am grateful for:

SATURDAY

SELF-CARE	MEAL PLAN	BODY MOVEMENT

Z^zz

Today I am grateful for:

SUNDAY

SELF-CARE	MEAL PLAN	BODY MOVEMENT

Z^zz

Today I am grateful for:

The endocrine system, also known as the hormonal system, consists of all the glands that produce and secrete hormones. The endocrine system is incredibly important because it affects every part of your body. Keeping it balanced is one of the keys to health.

Right now, my relationship with myself feels . . .

How to track your cycle

Okay ... so we now know about the incredible amount of change going on internally during our cycle ... it's time to understand how to recognise and track these changes by listening to the messages our body sends us each and every day.

The menstrual cycle gives you an opportunity to gain insight into your health. The info you gain from tracking your cycle can help you to either conceive a baby or avoid conceiving a baby.

Tracking and understanding your cycle can show you when you are fertile and ovulating. And using that knowledge to determine when to have or avoid sex is a type of contraception known as the Fertility Awareness Method (FAM). When used correctly, FAM is 99.4% effective and when used typically, it is 98.2% effective.

Tracking your cycle isn't just helpful for contraception or conception though. It can also help you to connect with your body and understand how your body shows up in the different phases of your cycle.

WHAT DOES A TYPICAL CYCLE LOOK LIKE?

* Begins day 1 of your period
* Cycle about 28 to 35 days long
* Period about 3 to 7 days long
* Ovulation around day 14
* Period about 14 days after ovulation

If you have a cycle that is longer than what's noted above, your body may be having difficulty ovulating. And if it's shorter, your body may not be producing normal levels of an important hormone called progesterone.

If your cycle differs from the above, talk to your health practitioner about it.

UNDERSTANDING YOUR CYCLE

Using the Cycle Chart that can be found in the monthly charts section of your journal (see page 233), track the following features to gain a thorough understanding of your cycle.

The date your period begins and ends

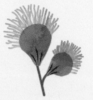

* Take notice if your period is long, heavy or painful. Although common, long, heavy, painful periods aren't optimal and they can indicate that something else is going on.

Your cervical fluid (also known as cervical mucous [CM] or discharge)

* Check your underwear and toilet paper for the consistency of your cervical fluid. Or if there's not much showing up, you can use clean fingers to check internally in your vagina. This might seem gross to do, but we have just been conditioned to think this! Our cervical fluid provides so much insight – we should 100% be taught this info at school.
* The consistency reflects how fertile you are at the time:
    · Technically, all cervical fluid can be fertile. But it becomes more fertile the closer you are to ovulation and the fluid's consistency reflects this.
    · Sticky fluid is not very fertile.
    · Creamy fluid is somewhat fertile.
    · Watery fluid is quite fertile.
    · Raw egg white fluid is very fertile and indicates your most fertile time – you are likely ovulating or going to ovulate within the next 72 hours.
    · In a typical cycle, after your period ends, your cervical fluid will turn creamy, watery then egg white in the lead-up to ovulation. After ovulation and in the lead-up to your next period, you may have sticky cervical fluid or not much cervical fluid.
    · Take note if there is not much cervical fluid all cycle. This can indicate low estrogen.
    · Also notice if your cervical fluid seems to cycle through the different types over and over again, and you have a long cycle. This can indicate you are struggling to ovulate.

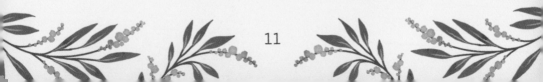

Cervical texture and position

* You can check your cervix by inserting clean fingers into your vagina.
* You will find your cervix by feeling towards the top of your vagina for something that feels round with a small indented hole in the centre, like a doughnut. You can check for the following:
  * Cervical position: is your cervix low in your vagina, or high?
  * Cervical texture: is your cervix feeling soft like your lips, or firm like the tip of your nose?
  * A soft cervical texture combined with a high cervical position indicates that you may be ovulating.

Basal body temperature (BBT)

* This can indicate your level of progesterone and therefore if you have ovulated. Progesterone and BBT often dip just before ovulation then rise once ovulation has occurred. They will stay high until you get your period, when they will drop. Or, if you are pregnant, they will remain high.
* Your BBT can be taken using a BBT thermometer. This is a thermometer that measures to two decimal places (e.g. 36.83 rather than 36.8).
* Measure your BBT as soon as you wake up, before getting out of bed or eating or drinking.
* Measure your BBT at the same time every day.
* Although your BBT is useful information for retrospectively understanding if and when you have ovulated, it is no longer seen as a good tool for knowing when you are currently ovulating. This is because it has now been found that not all people have a dip in progesterone and temperature just before ovulation. And, the rise in progesterone and temperature usually occurs *after* ovulation, when it is then too late to do anything about it as you have already ovulated and your fertile window has closed.

* Tracking your BBT is a *fantastic* way of knowing if you have actually ovulated and if you have good progesterone levels. If your temperature doesn't rise, even though it seems you have ovulated, and you get a period about 14 days after you think you have ovulated, it may indicate that you actually haven't ovulated at all (known as an anovulatory cycle) and the bleed is actually occurring because your body's progesterone levels are low. This can happen when your prolactin is high. It is very helpful information for your health practitioner and you should definitely let them know about it so they can test your prolactin and progesterone levels.

If you're having trouble conceiving, it can be a good idea to do the things listed above that you feel comfortable with to get some more insight into what might be happening. And if you're not trying to conceive but want to understand where you're at, give it a go – even just for one cycle. If you're interested in using the FAM method for contraception, really get to understand the method, do some extra reading if need be, and even consider booking an appointment with a fertility awareness educator.

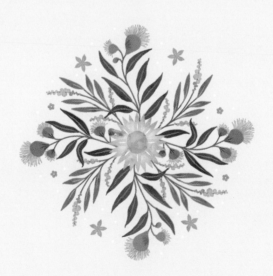

Intention for the week:

MONDAY

SELF-CARE	MEAL PLAN	BODY MOVEMENT
Zᶻᶻ		

Today I am grateful for:

TUESDAY

SELF-CARE	MEAL PLAN	BODY MOVEMENT
Zᶻᶻ		

Today I am grateful for:

WEDNESDAY

SELF-CARE	MEAL PLAN	BODY MOVEMENT
Zᶻᶻ		

Today I am grateful for:

THURSDAY

SELF-CARE	MEAL PLAN	BODY MOVEMENT
Zᶻᶻ		

Today I am grateful for:

Low estrogen can cause vaginal dryness, difficulties ovulating and conceiving, fatigue, dry skin and hair loss. Estrogen levels can be tested with a simple blood test and a practitioner may use spearmint tea, dong quai or diindolylmethane (DIM) to increase levels.

FRIDAY

SELF-CARE	MEAL PLAN	BODY MOVEMENT

Zᶻᶻ

Today I am grateful for:

SATURDAY

SELF-CARE	MEAL PLAN	BODY MOVEMENT

Zᶻᶻ

Today I am grateful for:

SUNDAY

SELF-CARE	MEAL PLAN	BODY MOVEMENT

Zᶻᶻ

Today I am grateful for:

The everyday pressures of life (and any hormonal imbalances that might go with it) can sometimes make us moody and temperamental. If this is affecting your relationships, try to embrace the simple but often forgotten concept of being kind. When brought to the forefront of our minds, kindness can wrap ease and respect around every thought we think and every sentence we speak.

What matters most in my life?

Welcome to Anatomy 101...

Minus the awkward teacher and all that *pussy*footing. See what we did there? Here we have a diagram of the reproductive system. You've probably seen it before ... but have you ever marvelled at that thing? The uterus is usually no bigger than a pear but at full-term pregnancy, it can be as big as a watermelon. Superhero stretchiness aside, the uterus is the *strongest* muscle in our body.

We've also got a diagram of the (oft-forgotten-by-sex-ed-teachers) vulva.

We'd love to know if you were today-years-old when you discovered that the exposed part of your reproductive organs was called the vulva, not the vagina.

One last thing – there is no such thing as a 'standard-looking' vulva. The only thing that's standard is that your vulva probably looks different from your friend's vulva. Vulvas are unique and every one of them is glorious.

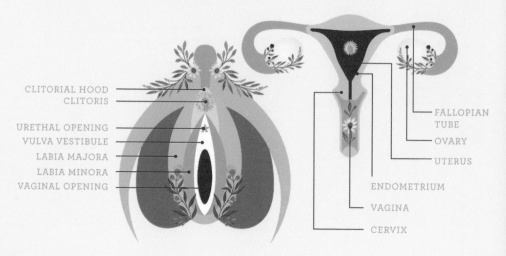

The whole body is connected

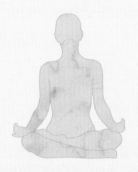

From the brain to the thyroid, gut and uterus; from our emotions to our immune system, skin and physical pain – it is all connected. Not just in an airy kind of way. In a biochemical, physiological way.

Until about 300 years ago, the mind and body were treated as one entity. Western medicine deviated from this and began to treat them as two separate systems, but most other medical modalities existing in the world still see the mind and body as connected.

And research is increasingly showing just how connected the mind and body is. The stress you feel is just as powerful for your physical health as the food you eat.

Stress can directly impact our immune system and potentially cause physical pain in our body, thyroid issues, digestive issues, reproductive issues, and issues with fatigue, memory and mental health.

The same could be said of our gut health, which can affect every facet of our body – including our mental health and happy hormones such as serotonin.

It is all connected.

If something does go out of balance and you find yourself with symptoms or a diagnosis of some kind, it is all about listening to your body, finding support, getting thorough testing, and finding and addressing the root cause.

Research is showing that thorough health care means our health professionals need to see the body as a whole, not in separate parts.

If a part of your body needs help, the entire body and mind should be considered.

Intention for the week:

MONDAY

SELF-CARE	MEAL PLAN	BODY MOVEMENT

Z^z_z

Today I am grateful for:

TUESDAY

SELF-CARE	MEAL PLAN	BODY MOVEMENT

Z^z_z

Today I am grateful for:

WEDNESDAY

SELF-CARE	MEAL PLAN	BODY MOVEMENT

Z^z_z

Today I am grateful for:

THURSDAY

SELF-CARE	MEAL PLAN	BODY MOVEMENT

Z^z_z

Today I am grateful for:

Healthy words:

I deeply and completely love, respect, appreciate and accept myself.

FRIDAY

SELF-CARE	MEAL PLAN	BODY MOVEMENT

Z^z_z

Today I am grateful for:

SATURDAY

SELF-CARE	MEAL PLAN	BODY MOVEMENT

Z^z_z

Today I am grateful for:

SUNDAY

SELF-CARE	MEAL PLAN	BODY MOVEMENT

Z^z_z

Today I am grateful for:

When you're struggling with symptoms, it can be easy to see your body as your enemy. But symptoms are your body's way of communicating with you that something is up. So take your body, pull it over to you so you're on the same team, and work together to investigate your symptoms and solve what's going on.

What is something you can do for yourself today to nurture your health?

The truth about the pill

I f you can't tell from the content we've already shared in this journal, your hormones are a super-delicate and important element of your health.

So helping you to understand the effect hormonal birth control has on your hormones is essential. It is fundamental information for all people.

Hormonal birth control – usually 'the pill' – is prescribed to people as a matter of course, for many reasons other than birth control.

Period pain, irregular periods, hormonal imbalances, acne, PMS – the first thing offered is often the pill. But the truth is, the pill is a band-aid solution for these issues. And it comes with a massive list of side effects that are less rare than you think. In fact, many are common.

And that period you get when on the pill? It isn't actually a period at all – it's a withdrawal bleed that happens when you take the sugar pills and your body withdraws from the steroid hormones in the regular pills.

The way the pill works is by shutting down your body's production of hormones such as progesterone, estrogen, luteinising hormone and follicle-stimulating hormone, so you don't ovulate. That's why it's so effective as a contraceptive.

But when we lose those powerful hormones, we lose all the benefits that come with them. These hormones are a lens through which we experience life. They help us to feel happy, vibrant, attractive and creative. They even help our brain function better and protect us from health conditions such as osteoporosis.

So when we take the pill or any other hormonal birth control, we not only increase our risk of a massive range of symptoms and conditions that can present themselves both while taking them and also after ceasing them, we also risk changing our entire experience of life.

When we think of it this way, it's no wonder that hormonal birth control can cause depression and anxiety for many of the people taking it.

And what about the expectation that we will take it?

To prevent making a baby, can you imagine a world in which society or the medical community would encourage a cis man to take a drug that completely shuts down his production of testosterone? Can you imagine many cis men in your life who would do that?

People have every right to choose to be on the pill for its band-aid benefits (for extreme pain that can be felt in conditions like endometriosis, the pill can be a great solution) and its excellent contraceptive effects – but it is unethical and goes against our health rights that people are prescribed the pill without all the info. This is not informed consent.

In lieu of our doctors being taught to share this info with us, please consider the side effects listed below and make an informed decision about whether or not the pill or any other hormonal contraceptive is right for you.

SYMPTOMS AND CONDITIONS THE PILL INCREASES YOUR RISK OF:

* Cervical cancer
* Breast cancer
* Post-birth-control syndrome (see page 68)
* Brain tumours
* Blood clots
* Heart attack
* Stroke
* Low libido
* Fertility issues
* Weight gain
* Anxiety and depression
* Irritable bowel syndrome (IBS)
* Hair loss
* Fatigue
* Inflammation
* Acne
* Extreme mood swings
* Suicidal ideation and suicide
* Nutrient deficiency

This information needs to be known by everyone. Too many people suffer because of hormonal birth control and the only way to change this is by spreading the knowledge. Many of our doctors are often in the dark about this too – their understanding of the matter is sometimes incomplete. So tell your friends, your sisters, your mothers, your daughters, your girlfriends *and* your doctors. And while you're at it, tell the cis men in your life – contraception and the health of the people in their life taking hormonal contraceptives are their issues too.

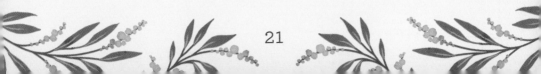

Intention for the week:

MONDAY

SELF-CARE

MEAL PLAN

BODY MOVEMENT

Z^z_z

Today I am grateful for:

TUESDAY

SELF-CARE

MEAL PLAN

BODY MOVEMENT

Z^z_z

Today I am grateful for:

WEDNESDAY

SELF-CARE

MEAL PLAN

BODY MOVEMENT

Z^z_z

Today I am grateful for:

THURSDAY

SELF-CARE

MEAL PLAN

BODY MOVEMENT

Z^z_z

Today I am grateful for:

Taking the birth control pill can deplete your body of important nutrients. This can potentially cause deficiencies in zinc, vitamin C, vitamin E, magnesium, folate, B2, B6, B12 and selenium.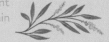

FRIDAY

SELF-CARE	MEAL PLAN	BODY MOVEMENT

Zᶻᶻ

Today I am grateful for:

SATURDAY

SELF-CARE	MEAL PLAN	BODY MOVEMENT

Zᶻᶻ

Today I am grateful for:

SUNDAY

SELF-CARE	MEAL PLAN	BODY MOVEMENT

Zᶻᶻ

Today I am grateful for:

Progesterone does more than just play an important role in reproduction. When progesterone surges after ovulation, it can make you feel happier and calmer, and can reduce anxiety. Progesterone is also anti-inflammatory and helps your hair and nails grow. When you use hormonal birth control, you produce zero progesterone.

Three things I love about myself are . . .

Birth control options
that won't mess with your hormones

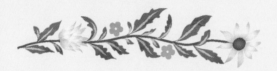

Whether it's the pill, hormonal IUD, implant, ring, patch or depo – hormonal birth control options shut down your own hormone production and come with a huge range of side effects.

So we need some alternatives, right? We can't leave you high and dry! Or wet, as the case may be . . .

If you're looking for birth control options that won't mess with your hormones, consider the following:

Condoms

* 98% effective with perfect use
* Trusty, effective and come with the added benefit of protecting you from sexually transmitted infections (STIs)
* Not always available and can break

Fertility Awareness Method (FAM)

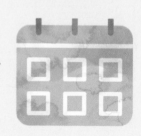

* 99.4%–99.6% effective with perfect use
* Helps you connect with and understand your body, cycle and hormones
* Takes time to learn

Copper IUD

* 99.4% effective
* Long-term contraception that doesn't prevent ovulation but instead works by creating an uninhabitable environment for the sperm and egg
* Painful to have inserted and comes with some serious potential side effects such as depression, bacterial vaginosis and uterine perforation

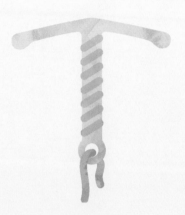

Diaphragm

* 94% effective with perfect use
* No need to rely on the person with the penis in the room and is fairly easy to use
* Requires spermicide each time it is used and can cause discomfort

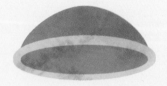

Withdrawal method

* 96% effective with perfect use
* Can be done anywhere and at any time
* Substantial pregnancy risk when not done properly and relies on the person with the penis

Intention for the week:

MONDAY

SELF-CARE   MEAL PLAN   BODY MOVEMENT

Z^z_z

Today I am grateful for:

TUESDAY

SELF-CARE   MEAL PLAN   BODY MOVEMENT

Z^z_z

Today I am grateful for:

WEDNESDAY

SELF-CARE   MEAL PLAN   BODY MOVEMENT

Z^z_z

Today I am grateful for:

THURSDAY

SELF-CARE   MEAL PLAN   BODY MOVEMENT

Z^z_z

Today I am grateful for:

'Here's to strong women. May we know them. May we be them. May we raise them' – UNKNOWN

FRIDAY

SELF-CARE	MEAL PLAN	BODY MOVEMENT

Z^z_z

Today I am grateful for:

SATURDAY

SELF-CARE	MEAL PLAN	BODY MOVEMENT

Z^z_z

Today I am grateful for:

SUNDAY

SELF-CARE	MEAL PLAN	BODY MOVEMENT

Z^z_z

Today I am grateful for:

Estrogen does more than just play an important role in reproduction. The main estrogen we produce is estradiol. It slows the aging process, raises libido and increases levels of serotonin, which is important for mood and sleep. When you use hormonal birth control, you produce zero estradiol.

This week, I loved seeing . . . .

Let's reflect on those basics

I n this chapter, you've learnt the fundamental things you need to understand to be able to utilise your journal to its maximum capability. And you've learnt things that are essential knowledge for all people.

At the end of each chapter, you will find a reflection page like this to help you understand how your new knowledge can play a role in your life.

Will you be tracking your cycle from here on in?
☐ Oh 100% ☐ Nah

Is the FAM method a contraceptive approach that you would consider using?
☐ Yes! ☐ Already using it ☐ Not for me

Does your cycle fit the parameters of what is 'typical'?
☐ Looks like it! ☐ Eek ... maybe not and I'm going to talk to my health practitioner about it.

Let's look at your cervical fluid! What does it look like today?
☐ Creamy ☐ Watery ☐ Clear egg white ☐ Sticky ☐ None

What quantity of cervical fluid do you normally see?

Okay ... did you know your vulva was called a vulva?!
☐ Duh! ☐ No! Can't wait to start referring to it correctly
☐ Nah babe, that thing will be called a vagina forevermore

Does understanding the risks associated with hormonal birth control change anything for you?
☐ Nope – I love the benefits ☐ I was never interested in using it anyway
☐ I'm going to find a new solution ☐ I won't be using hormonal birth control in the future

Do you think you will share what you've learnt about hormonal birth control with your people?
☐ 100% – they need to know! ☐ I'm not sure? ☐ Nah ... not my thing

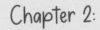

Chapter 2

CAN WE GET A LITTLE SUPPORT UP IN HERE?

Sure, this journal is going to make you about 478 times wiser . . . but at the end of the day, although you are the wise ruler of your body, a wise ruler still needs wise advisers.

When it comes to your health, advisers come in the form of health practitioners.

There are some incredible health practitioners out there. Health practitioners who are curious, kind, invested in your health and who listen.

But here's the thing – you need advisers you can trust and respect . . . but you also need advisers who trust and respect *you*. Because ultimately, rulers run things, not advisers.

But . . . a ruler without advisers can become truly lost, especially if any tricky challenges come their way.

And that's why this chapter is going to help you understand the kinds of health practitioners who exist to advise you, and what to look for in a health practitioner.

To start with, we want you to understand a term that has finally emerged, which describes what so many of us find ourselves struggling with.

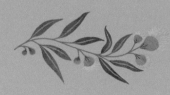

Medical gaslighting . . . yep, it's a thing

But don't worry, we're not powerless and we can do something about it. In recent years, you may have heard of the term *gaslighting*. Gaslighting is a form of psychological abuse where a person or group makes someone question their sanity, perception of reality or memories. It's often talked about in the context of relationships.

It is a fantastic term that has given language to people worldwide to help them voice their experiences, concerns and abuse.

What hasn't been talked about enough, though, is that gaslighting happens in a medical setting too, and it can have a devastating impact.

Medical gaslighting occurs when a health professional downplays or explains away symptoms or concerns with non-medical or psychological reasons, or they deny the concern completely, or try and convince you that you're imagining it. Examples:

* Telling your doctor you are getting stomach pain every day and them dismissing it as anxiety.
* Showing concern about a physical symptom and them asking if you've been under a lot of stress lately.
* Ridicule or amusement in response to your concerns.
* Having concerns about something you read on Google that resonated with you, and them dismissing you because you read it on Google.
* Presenting with extreme period pain and being dismissed because 'people just get period pain'.
* Being made to feel like the symptoms you're experiencing aren't as painful, intense or frequent as you think they are.

Gaslighting can lead patients to doubt themselves, feel like they're overreacting, or question their own memory and sanity. This can result in increased and prolonged pain, and incorrect or underdiagnosis, which can put lives at risk.

It has been found that medical gaslighting is more likely to be experienced by women and in illnesses that don't yet have a clear diagnostic test, for example, chronic fatigue syndrome and endometriosis.

It is reported that it can take up to 12 years for people to be diagnosed with endometriosis. Similar statistics can be found in people with polycystic ovarian syndrome (PCOS) – up to 70% of which goes undiagnosed. Heart disease is the leading cause of death in women, yet it has been found that women are prescribed less medicine and offered surgery less often than men. Studies have also found that women are less likely to receive treatment for conditions ranging from strokes to knee pain, with one study finding that when women present to the emergency room with stomach pain, they will wait 65 minutes to get help versus the 49 minutes it takes for men to receive pain relief.

Doctors don't always know they are gaslighting. It has been found that they can have biases that they are unaware of.

But a good doctor should be warm, interested and engaged; should take the time to make you feel comfortable; and should listen to and recognise your concerns.

WHAT CAN YOU DO TO AVOID MEDICAL GASLIGHTING?

No-one can completely understand what it feels like to go through all that *you* go through with your health – so it's up to you to be your best advocate. That doesn't mean you don't need a doctor. It means acknowledging that your health is your responsibility. Try the following:

1. **If your current doctor is gaslighting you, consider telling them.**
   Maybe start by insisting your concerns are real and you feel you're not being heard. If they still gaslight you, tell them it feels like they're gaslighting you. If doctors become aware of medical gaslighting, maybe they'll stop. It doesn't have to be confrontational. You could ask if they've heard the term and explain it feels like that's what is happening. If you can't get through to them, move on to step 2.

2. **Build an awesome healthcare team around you that you trust.** Don't be afraid to look outside of Western medicine or have a team of practitioners you can turn to – a GP for tests, Chinese medicine for acupuncture, Ayurveda for lifestyle advice . . . *you* are the ruler of your body and your health professionals are your advisers – there are good ones out there, we promise.

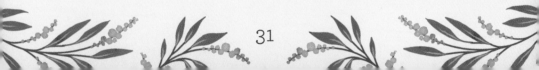

Intention for the week:

MONDAY

SELF-CARE	MEAL PLAN	BODY MOVEMENT

Z^z_z

Today I am grateful for:

TUESDAY

SELF-CARE	MEAL PLAN	BODY MOVEMENT

Z^z_z

Today I am grateful for:

WEDNESDAY

SELF-CARE	MEAL PLAN	BODY MOVEMENT

Z^z_z

Today I am grateful for:

THURSDAY

SELF-CARE	MEAL PLAN	BODY MOVEMENT

Z^z_z

Today I am grateful for:

Zinc is a nutrient that helps your immune system and metabolism function and can increase fertility; lower insulin levels; improve hirsutism, inflammation, hair loss, acne and PMS; and heal your gut.

FRIDAY

SELF-CARE	MEAL PLAN	BODY MOVEMENT

Z^z_z

Today I am grateful for:

SATURDAY

SELF-CARE	MEAL PLAN	BODY MOVEMENT

Z^z_z

Today I am grateful for:

SUNDAY

SELF-CARE	MEAL PLAN	BODY MOVEMENT

Z^z_z

Today I am grateful for:

Set time aside as often as you can to do something that steps you and your health forward. Give yourself a foot massage, book an appointment with that naturopath your friend recommended, go for a walk, cuddle a hot water bottle, make a cup of tea . . . give yourself the time to prioritise your health. You're using this journal because you want to be your healthiest self. This is a way you can begin to do that.

Right now, I feel like my lifestyle is . . .

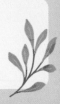

Things you're allowed to say to your doctor

After reading about medical gaslighting and finding great advisers for your health, you may be left wondering if your doctor is up to scratch. This week, we're looking at some of the things you are 100% allowed to say to your doctor. Keep this list in mind going forward and, hopefully, your confidence in your doctor can grow.

Remember, *you* hire your doctor. They work for *you*. And you can seek a new doctor any time you like.

- ✴ Are there any alternative treatment options?

- ✴ Please print a copy of my test results for me.

- ✴ Could I get your opinion on something I've read?

- ✴ I'm requesting this test because I'm concerned this is affecting me and I want to know for sure.

- ✴ Can you explain that further?

- ✴ If you haven't heard of this treatment/test, can you recommend a practitioner who might have?

- ✴ I'm passionate about my health and I need a doctor who accepts that I'm a part of the team. Are you open to that?

- ✴ I have a bunch of questions – can we go through them?

Functional medicine

Over the next few weeks, you will begin to learn about some effective, thorough and natural approaches to health. Often, consults with natural medicine practitioners are one to two hours long. Support like that is priceless and can lead to a deeper understanding of what could be affecting your health.

We're beginning with functional medicine – a relatively new practice that began in the 1990s and is largely focused on preventing and treating chronic illnesses, such as endometriosis, PCOS, diabetes, IBS and more. Its scientific model seeks to find the underlying cause of a person's illness by examining the processes that occur in the body along with the physiological, environmental and psychological factors of an individual.

Functional medicine practitioners do extensive testing of their patient's core systems, including the immune, gastrointestinal and endocrine (hormonal) systems, and use natural medicine, nutrition, lifestyle practices and pharmaceuticals (if necessary) to design a treatment plan tailored to their patient.

How researched is it? Fairly well. The testing used is completely science-based but the medicines vary. Many medicines are heavily researched but because natural medicines are also used, some may not be as researched as others – as is found with any natural medicine practice.

Is it for you? If you're interested in understanding the deep functioning of your body or in discovering the possible cause of your chronic illness, then it's for you.

How accessible is it? Functional medicine is growing in popularity with some practitioners believing it is the future of medicine. You may however have trouble finding it outside of the Western world. Also, although the consultations may be cost-effective, the testing you may be encouraged to do can be costly.

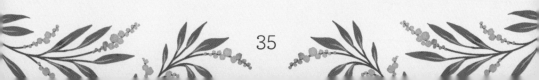

WEEK 7

Intention for the week:

MONDAY

SELF-CARE	MEAL PLAN	BODY MOVEMENT
Zᶻz		

Today I am grateful for:

TUESDAY

SELF-CARE	MEAL PLAN	BODY MOVEMENT
Zᶻz		

Today I am grateful for:

WEDNESDAY

SELF-CARE	MEAL PLAN	BODY MOVEMENT
Zᶻz		

Today I am grateful for:

THURSDAY

SELF-CARE	MEAL PLAN	BODY MOVEMENT
Zᶻz		

Today I am grateful for:

Healthy words:

I am healthy, happy and radiant.

FRIDAY

SELF-CARE	MEAL PLAN	BODY MOVEMENT

Z^z_z

Today I am grateful for:

SATURDAY

SELF-CARE	MEAL PLAN	BODY MOVEMENT

Z^z_z

Today I am grateful for:

SUNDAY

SELF-CARE	MEAL PLAN	BODY MOVEMENT

Z^z_z

Today I am grateful for:

Research has shown that about 40% of people between the ages of 26 and 83 have low levels of vitamin B12. Low levels of B12 are linked to many symptoms including infertility, fatigue, difficulty metabolising carbohydrates and irrational anger.

Something I love about my body is . . .

Ayurveda

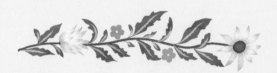

Thought to be more than 5,000 years old, Ayurveda (eye-er-vae-duh) is the world's oldest practising medical system. Ayurveda originated in India and translates as the 'science of life'. It is considered a base of wisdom to help people lead vibrant, healthy lives while embracing all they are capable of.

One of the main guiding principles of Ayurveda is that the mind, body and spirit are inextricably connected, and that to prevent and treat disease, each (and the connection between them) must be nourished. This is done through nutrition, lifestyle practices, panchakarma (detoxifying treatments), herbal medicine, yoga asanas (poses), pranayama (deep breathing), mudras (hand gestures), mantra, massage, meditation and aromatherapy.

The Ayurvedic practice teaches that five elements – earth, water, fire, air and space – make up the human body and everything in the universe. It is believed we are each born with a unique combination of these elements that form our balanced place. The word 'dosha' describes how these elements function within us. There are three main doshas – vata, pitta and kapha.

VATA	PITTA	KAPHA
Primarily space and air	Primarily fire and water	Primarily water and earth
Thin and bony	Moderate build & muscular limbs	Broad frames and long limbs
Restless mind	Alert mind	Calm and patient

Ayurvedic practitioners assess your constitution and state of imbalance by asking you a series of questions, so they can create a personalised treatment plan for you based on your constitution and the symptoms you are presenting with.

It all might sound strange but it is a truly effective practice that produces fantastic results for many people.

How researched is it? Somewhat – high-quality research is certainly still needed. However, there are an increasing number of studies showing how effective it is. What also shouldn't be ignored are the countless testimonials from people who have had incredible results. And with its thousands of years of practice and refinement, it is considered so effective a medical system that it is still practised alongside Western medicine in hospitals throughout India.

Is it for you? If the idea of the mind-body connection speaks to you, and if you read about the doshas and felt like you were reading about yourself – it could be for you. If you have tried other options and you are still searching for the right treatment path for you, then every treatment option is a possible way forward – Ayurveda is as valid an option as any.

How accessible is it? Fairly. If you are living in southern Asia or in a city or large town anywhere in the world it should be easy to find an Ayurvedic practitioner. However, if you live in a small regional area outside of southern Asia, you may have difficulty. There are many practitioners online.

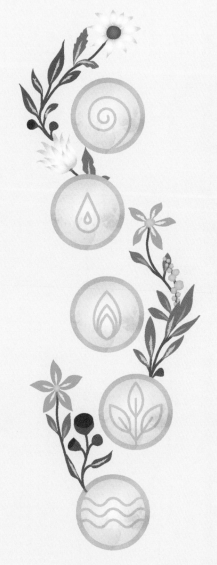

WEEK 8

Intention for the week:

MONDAY

SELF-CARE	MEAL PLAN	BODY MOVEMENT

Z^z_z

Today I am grateful for:

TUESDAY

SELF-CARE	MEAL PLAN	BODY MOVEMENT

Z^z_z

Today I am grateful for:

WEDNESDAY

SELF-CARE	MEAL PLAN	BODY MOVEMENT

Z^z_z

Today I am grateful for:

THURSDAY

SELF-CARE	MEAL PLAN	BODY MOVEMENT

Z^z_z

Today I am grateful for:

Karavellaka is a bitter fruit used in Ayurveda that can regulate your period, reduce inflammation and assist in weight loss.

FRIDAY

SELF-CARE	MEAL PLAN	BODY MOVEMENT
Zᶻᶻ		

Today I am grateful for:

SATURDAY

SELF-CARE	MEAL PLAN	BODY MOVEMENT
Zᶻᶻ		

Today I am grateful for:

SUNDAY

SELF-CARE	MEAL PLAN	BODY MOVEMENT
Zᶻᶻ		

Today I am grateful for:

In Ayurveda, the day is broken into 4-hour blocks, each governed by a specific dosha. It is encouraged to align your life with these cycles of nature. 6–10 am/pm = kapha, a grounding time to be introspective and nurturing. 10–2 am/pm = pitta, a time of energy to get things done, have your largest meal of the day and process at night. 2–6 am/pm = vata, a time of transition to socialise, create and explore spiritual practices.

Something healthy that makes me feel great is . . .

Naturopathy

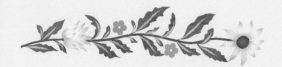

Naturopathy is the practice of natural medicine. It encompasses the use of Western herbal medicine (the most widely practised medical system in the world), vitamins, minerals, amino acids, massage, and dietary and lifestyle practices to prevent and treat disease.

It is a powerful approach that offers a large range of treatment options for most health issues. Even when Western medicine is the best option – for example, in the case of surgery or heart disease – naturopathy offers treatments that can complement and improve your outcomes.

Naturopathy is practised in varying ways by naturopaths, homeopaths and herbalists, and almost always accompanies recommendations for the ideal diet, exercise and lifestyle for *your* body.

A naturopathic practitioner will assess your body and your symptoms to create a tailored treatment program that suits you. Many will also support you in asking your doctor for relevant blood tests, which will help the naturopathic practitioner understand your body and treat it appropriately.

One thing that is fantastic about naturopathic practitioners is that they tend to look at your test results a bit more deeply than a doctor might. For example, if your blood test results for zinc sit low within the 'normal range', many doctors would probably say that there is no issue. A naturopathic practitioner, however, often takes the time to consider if low zinc could have a part to play in your symptoms and decide if zinc supplementation could help you.

How researched is it? Many naturopathic medicines have been extensively researched (although many have not and are used based more upon clinical evidence).

Is it for you? If you are after a well-researched practice that uses natural medicine, naturopathy could be perfect for you. If you have a health condition and feel you have run out of options, but haven't seen a naturopathic practitioner – consider booking an appointment. You may just find exactly the treatment you need.

How accessible is it? Naturopathic practitioners can be found worldwide, even remotely.

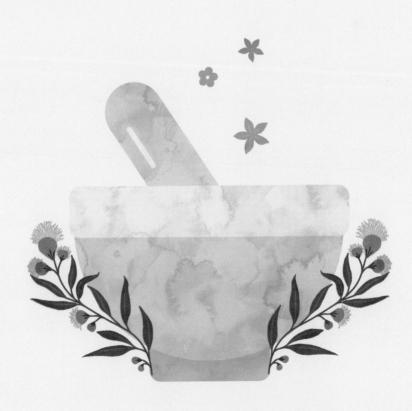

WEEK 9

Intention for the week:

MONDAY
SELF-CARE | MEAL PLAN | BODY MOVEMENT

Zᶻᶻ

Today I am grateful for:

TUESDAY
SELF-CARE | MEAL PLAN | BODY MOVEMENT

Zᶻᶻ

Today I am grateful for:

WEDNESDAY
SELF-CARE | MEAL PLAN | BODY MOVEMENT

Zᶻᶻ

Today I am grateful for:

THURSDAY
SELF-CARE | MEAL PLAN | BODY MOVEMENT

Zᶻᶻ

Today I am grateful for:

'A person who has good thoughts cannot ever be ugly. You can have a wonky nose and a crooked mouth and a double chin and stick-out teeth, but if you have good thoughts they will shine out of your face like sunbeams and you will always look lovely.' – ROALD DAHL, THE TWITS

FRIDAY

SELF-CARE	MEAL PLAN	BODY MOVEMENT

Z^z_z

Today I am grateful for:

SATURDAY

SELF-CARE	MEAL PLAN	BODY MOVEMENT

Z^z_z

Today I am grateful for:

SUNDAY

SELF-CARE	MEAL PLAN	BODY MOVEMENT

Z^z_z

Today I am grateful for:

It is estimated that 80% of people are magnesium deficient due to the decreased quality of our soil. Magnesium can improve sugar metabolism, sleep and period pain, calm the nervous system, support thyroid hormones and increase energy, serotonin and dopamine. You can support magnesium levels with a magnesium supplement, magnesium spray or magnesium salt bath.

A perfect day looks like . . .

Traditional Chinese medicine

Originating in ancient China, traditional Chinese medicine (TCM) has been practised for about 2,500 years. It is built on the ancient belief that health is achieved when there is a balance between the two opposing forces of yin and yang, allowing easy movement of qi (vital energy) throughout the body. It is believed that an imbalance of yin and yang results in disease.

TCM has a focus on prevention over treatment but can help no matter where you are on your health journey. The number of herbal options offered by TCM is incredible. If you feel you have 'tried everything' and yet you haven't tried TCM, then get excited because TCM is a whole world of options.

WHAT TECHNIQUES ARE USED IN TCM?

TCM uses herbal medicine, acupuncture, qi gong (a form of exercise), massage, cupping, gua sha, moxibustion, nutrition and lifestyle practices.

How researched is it? Many herbs and practices used in TCM have been researched but continued research is still needed. TCM can be difficult to assess in clinical trials because the combination of herbs used is so tailored to the individual. What should be considered though are the thousands of years of practice, refinement and clinical evidence, along with the countless anecdotal testimonials from patients who have had positive results.

Is it for you? If you are someone who can connect with the idea of an energetic system and yin and yang – balance – then TCM is right up your alley. TCM is a complete system of medicine backed by thousands of years of empirical evidence as well as modern research – it's as valid an option as any.

How accessible is it? TCM is prolific throughout the world. If relevant, try to find a practitioner with a focused interest in your particular health concern.

Other modalities to consider

So far we have looked at some complete medical systems that are widely accepted and can really tackle most symptoms and conditions. But there are so many more modalities out there that can support you in various ways on your health journey.

Here is a list of some popular standouts and what they do.

* **Dietetics:** the understood science of how food and nutrition react in the body and affect our health. Dietitians can help people with any nutritional issues they have. **How supported by science?** Super supported by science.

* **Kinesiology:** the study of body movements. Kinesiologists use muscle monitoring to locate and correct imbalances in the body. Practitioners use kinesiology to heal physical, emotional and spiritual issues. **How supported by science?** Mildly. The practice isn't scientifically proven as a concept, but studies show it can be effective.

* **Reflexology:** based on the theory that by stimulating areas on the feet with specific pressure techniques, the body's natural healing mechanism can be activated. **How supported by science?** Mildly. The concept of reflexology isn't scientifically proven, but studies show it can be effective.

* **Homeopathy:** based on the belief that the body can heal itself. Practitioners use highly diluted substances that can create similar symptoms to what you are experiencing because they believe it can stimulate the body's healing response. **How supported by science?** Mildly. The concept of homeopathy isn't scientifically proven, but studies show it can be effective.

* **Reiki:** a Japanese form of energy healing that is said to relieve stress and induce relaxation and healing. Practitioners use their hands to guide universal energy through the body. **How supported by science?** Mildly. The concept of reiki isn't scientifically proven, but studies show it can be effective.

Intention for the week:

MONDAY

SELF-CARE	MEAL PLAN	BODY MOVEMENT

Z^z_z

Today I am grateful for:

TUESDAY

SELF-CARE	MEAL PLAN	BODY MOVEMENT

Z^z_z

Today I am grateful for:

WEDNESDAY

SELF-CARE	MEAL PLAN	BODY MOVEMENT

Z^z_z

Today I am grateful for:

THURSDAY

SELF-CARE	MEAL PLAN	BODY MOVEMENT

Z^z_z

Today I am grateful for:

Used in TCM, berberine is a powerful herb that has been shown to reduce insulin resistance, improve gut health, reduce testosterone and aid in weight loss.

FRIDAY

SELF-CARE	MEAL PLAN	BODY MOVEMENT

Z^z_z

Today I am grateful for:

SATURDAY

SELF-CARE	MEAL PLAN	BODY MOVEMENT

Z^z_z

Today I am grateful for:

SUNDAY

SELF-CARE	MEAL PLAN	BODY MOVEMENT

Z^z_z

Today I am grateful for:

Studies have found that acupuncture can decrease luteinising hormone and testosterone, and improve insulin sensitivity. It has also been found to be an effective treatment for pain and nausea, and is used effectively for a wide range of conditions.

Who is someone you love who you haven't spoken to in ages? Maybe you could get in touch with them this week . . .

Let's reflect on that whole support thing

So, first things first . . . are you feeling like you're responsible for your own health?
- [ ] 100%
- [ ] It's a shift but I'm getting there
- [ ] I just want to lie down and put my health into someone else's hands

Do you currently have a great health practitioner?
- [ ] Yes, they're the best!
- [ ] I need to see them through new eyes at my next appointment
- [ ] No, they need to go and I need to find someone new

If you are in need of a new practitioner, what qualities are you hoping they will have?

_____

_____

_____

Have you experienced medical gaslighting?
- [ ] Yes
- [ ] I'm not sure
- [ ] No

How does it make you feel knowing that medical gaslighting exists?

_____

_____

_____

Is there a new modality of medicine you would like to explore?

_____

_____

_____

Do you feel more empowered to advocate for yourself?
- [ ] Definitely
- [ ] Already empowered, baby!

Chapter 3

PERIODS AND HORMONES AND CYCLES – OH MY!

We believe the disconnect many of us have with our body and our cycle is, at least in part, due to living in a patriarchal society. Whether at school, at home, in the workplace or in sporting activities, at some point you've probably been told you're being 'too hormonal' or 'too emotional'.

It's true – for some of us, our period comes with some annoying symptoms – we *can* feel more emotional. We can feel more pain, nausea and cravings.

The issue is we've been taught that these symptoms annoy people and are open to ridicule. This can lead to shame.

Periods make a lot of cis men squeamish. It's not a coincidence that we've been taught to keep our cycles private, push through the pain and show up 'like a man'. No wonder it takes people often upwards of 10 years to get a diagnosis of conditions that affect our period such as endometriosis and PCOS.

Our menstrual symptoms are messages from our body telling us about our internal health. Messages we've been taught to ignore or medicate so we can 'get on with things'. Learning to listen to these messages (and talk about them) will help shift our society beyond the patriarchy and into equality.

It's time people acknowledged that all humans have hormones and emotions, not just us. Testosterone is a hormone. Anger is an emotion. Isn't it interesting how that became ignored? In this chapter, we'll discover just how incredible each of our hormones are and how to understand and connect with our menstrual cycle so that we can thrive.

Phases of the menstrual cycle

One of the biggest disservices to people who get periods is the lack of education around the phases of the menstrual cycle. Our body is not the same day in and day out, and everyone should be taught that fact in school. This is a big issue that goes beyond how we experience our body and into how society and particularly work-culture is structured.

We are cyclical creatures but we are living in a static society, which we really didn't consent to because, historically, there was only one gender that had a say in it – cis men. The patriarchy. As we mentioned, a testosterone-based hormonal system is cyclical too – but the cycle is only 24 hours long. So every day, people with a testosterone-based hormonal system show up in pretty much the same way. And so, we've been expected to show up the same every day too – in our workplace, relationships, moods, emotions, physical ability . . . but our internal chemistry is not the same every single day.

The rise and fall of our hormones occurs over a much longer period of time – usually 25 to 35 *days* – and we have strengths that reveal themselves throughout that cycle. We have more energy at times, feel more confident at times, are more focused at times, and feel sexier, warmer and more nurturing at times.

Understanding the phases of your cycle can help you to connect with your body and can help you to know when to plan events and dates, when to harness your creativity and when to dive into that project you've been trying to get done.

The info below shares guidance for each phase of the cycle.

But this journal isn't just about guidance. It's about understanding *you*. We are all different and our cycles show up in different ways for all of us.

To understand the phases of your cycle, you need to look at the phases of *your* cycle. To help you with this, there is a chart in the monthly charts section (see page 308). Use it to record your experience of each phase of your cycle.

MENSTRUAL PHASE

Days: 1 up to 7 (typically)

Dominant hormone: follicle-stimulating hormone

Mood: Introverted, chilled, reflective, intuitive

Food: warm and easy to digest – soups, stews, slow cooked meat

Move: keep it gentle – rest, slow yoga, walking

Groove: creative, low energy, cleansing, home time, rest, quiet focus, reflection

FOLLICULAR PHASE

Days: end of period to whenever you ovulate

Dominant hormone: follicle stimulating hormone and estrogen

Mood: Energetic, vibrant, positive

Food: lighter foods with warm protein – balanced salads, sauteed greens, fruit salad

Move: Vigorous unless stressed or inflamed - cardio classes, bike riding, swimming

Groove: attend meetings, teamwork, problem solving, strategizing, starting projects

OVULATORY PHASE

Days: the day or two leading into ovulation

Dominant hormone: Luteinising hormone

Mood: confident, attractive, invincible

Food: raw and quick meals – salads, stir-fries, juices

Move: intense unless stressed or inflamed – HIIT, cross fit, running, dancing

Groove: social, public speaking, leading teams, negotiating deals, launching projects, making videos, networking, dating

LUTEAL PHASE

Days: ovulation to your period

Dominant hormone: progesterone

Mood: low energy, focused

Food: warm and comforting – roast veg, fish, wholegrains like rice, healthy fats like avocado

Move: light activity – short walks, relaxing swims, yoga, pilates, strength training

Groove: gentle, task oriented, attention to detail, admin tasks, bookkeeping, getting support and help, completing projects.

WEEK 11

Intention for the week:

MONDAY

SELF-CARE | MEAL PLAN | BODY MOVEMENT

Z^z_z

Today I am grateful for:

TUESDAY

SELF-CARE | MEAL PLAN | BODY MOVEMENT

Z^z_z

Today I am grateful for:

WEDNESDAY

SELF-CARE | MEAL PLAN | BODY MOVEMENT

Z^z_z

Today I am grateful for:

THURSDAY

SELF-CARE | MEAL PLAN | BODY MOVEMENT

Z^z_z

Today I am grateful for:

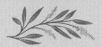

High in vitamin C and fibre, sprouts can help
remove excess hormones from the body.

FRIDAY

SELF-CARE	MEAL PLAN	BODY MOVEMENT

Z^z_z

Today I am grateful for:

SATURDAY

SELF-CARE	MEAL PLAN	BODY MOVEMENT

Z^z_z

Today I am grateful for:

SUNDAY

SELF-CARE	MEAL PLAN	BODY MOVEMENT

Z^z_z

Today I am grateful for:

There's a tendency to talk pretty negatively about periods. But your period is a sign that an important part of your body is functioning. If your period is bringing with it any kind of serious discomfort – this is a message from your body that something might be imbalanced. Try not to ignore or curse it. Try to listen to it, then talk to your doctor and address it.

This week, I feel proud of myself for . .

Signs your cycle is irregular . . .

and reasons it might be happening

Long, short, heavy, painful . . . so many people suffer silently with these symptoms because it can feel taboo to discuss periods . . . but this needs to end. Please chat to your health practitioner if you have any of these symptoms.

And for any teenagers reading this – know that in your teenage years a lot of this can actually be normal – to an extent. Your hormonal system is still developing and sorting itself out. If any of these symptoms are bothering you though, definitely bring it up with your health practitioner. And, anything more than mild period pain is always something to discuss with your doctor.

Long cycle (more than 35 days or 45 days in teenagers)

A long cycle means you're struggling to ovulate. Reasons include: polycystic ovarian syndrome (PCOS), hypothalamic amenorrhea, high prolactin, low estrogen, high androgens, elevated LH:FSH ratio, chronic stress, hypothyroidism, hyperthyroidism, celiac disease, under-eating and over-exercising.

Short cycle (less than 21 days)

Short cycles are usually anovulatory, meaning you haven't ovulated. Reasons include: low progesterone, perimenopause, hyperthyroidism, hypothyroidism, chronic stress and extreme weight fluctuations.

Short period

A period as short as one day can be considered normal if you have ovulated and if that's 'your normal'. If you haven't ovulated or if you are having unusually short periods for you, reasons include: progesterone, Asherman syndrome, under-eating, over-exercising, extreme weight loss, stress, some anti-inflammatory drugs, antidepressants, thyroid meds and steroids.

Long period (longer than 7 days)

If you have a long period, reasons include: endometriosis, anovulatory cycle, uterine fibroids, polyps, stagnation (a concept from Chinese medicine), pelvic inflammatory disease (PID), aspirin, perimenopause, underactive thyroid, liver or kidney disease, von Willebrand disease, cervical or uterine cancer.

Heavy, dark, clotting period

If you have a heavy, dark, clotting period, reasons include: high estrogen, anovulatory cycle, uterine fibroids, polyps, stagnation, PID, endometriosis, enlarged uterus, hypothyroidism, endometrial hyperplasia, adenomyosis, using anticoagulant drugs, liver or kidney disease, von Willebrand disease.

Period pain

If you have period pain, reasons include: stagnation, endometriosis, PID, uterine fibroids, polyps, adenomyosis, cervical stenosis, high levels of prostaglandins, Asherman's syndrome.

PMS

If you suffer from PMS, reasons include: brain sensitivity to changes in hormonal levels, hormonal imbalances, premenstrual dysmorphic disorder (not a cause of PMS but sometimes mistaken for PMS – see Chapter 5 for more info), low serotonin, smoking.

Mid-cycle spotting

If you have mid-cycle spotting, reasons include: ovulation spotting, PID, uterine fibroids, implantation bleeding, chlamydia, gonorrhoea, uterine or cervical cancer, sex, malnutrition, endometriosis, ovarian cysts, cervical ectropion, perimenopause and the morning-after pill.

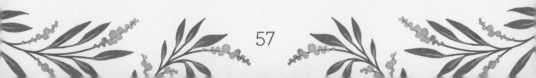

Intention for the week:

MONDAY

SELF-CARE	MEAL PLAN	BODY MOVEMENT

Z^z_z

Today I am grateful for:

TUESDAY

SELF-CARE	MEAL PLAN	BODY MOVEMENT

Z^z_z

Today I am grateful for:

WEDNESDAY

SELF-CARE	MEAL PLAN	BODY MOVEMENT

Z^z_z

Today I am grateful for:

THURSDAY

SELF-CARE	MEAL PLAN	BODY MOVEMENT

Z^z_z

Today I am grateful for:

Adenomyosis is a condition in which the tissue that lines the uterus grows into the muscle wall of the uterus, causing menstrual cramps, lower abdominal pressure, bloating and heavy periods.

FRIDAY

SELF-CARE	MEAL PLAN	BODY MOVEMENT

Z^z_z

Today I am grateful for:

SATURDAY

SELF-CARE	MEAL PLAN	BODY MOVEMENT

Z^z_z

Today I am grateful for:

SUNDAY

SELF-CARE	MEAL PLAN	BODY MOVEMENT

Z^z_z

Today I am grateful for:

How heavy is heavy? A period of more than 80 ml in total is classed as a heavy period. This is about 16 fully soaked regular tampons or eight fully soaked super tampons. If you are losing more blood than this, talk to your doctor about what might be causing it.

Am I taking anything for granted?

Get to know your flow

Did you know that the colour of your period blood can tell you things about your health?

It's just another example of our body constantly sending us information that we are usually blind to, because we are just not taught this info in school.

Take a photo of this page and take note next time you get your period!

Grey – not typical
Could mean:
* Bacterial vaginosis

Orange – possibly mixed with cervical fluid
Could mean:
* Possible infection

Pink – light coloured, watery
Could mean:
* Nutrient deficiency
* Anaemia
* Low estrogen
* Implantation bleeding

Bright red – fresh blood, smooth texture, steady flow
Could mean:
* A healthy period

Dark red – heavy, thick, clotting
Could mean:
* High estrogen
* Stagnation

Brown/rust – oxidised blood
Could mean:
* Too little progesterone
* Early sign of pregnancy
* Old blood moving out

Friendly alternatives to tampons

Okay, so now we know all about the colour of our period blood . . . what are we going to do with it? Thankfully, period products have evolved over the past decade.

Sure, tampons have served a purpose and for some, they're still the go-to.

But having options that are healthier for our body and for the planet is an example of the kind of progression we want to see.

Why wouldn't we want to use the trusty tampon?

* There are 20 *billion* disposable pads and tampons ending up in landfill every year . . . pretty wild for something we use for just a few hours.
* Tampons work by absorption, which can dry out and change the microbiome of your vagina, increasing your chance of infection.
* They can also cause toxic shock syndrome and cramping, and contain bleach and dioxins, which can cause cancer.
* Once disposed of, the chemicals in tampons soak into the earth, polluting our groundwater and air.
* Tampons are made from cotton, and growing cotton requires a vast amount of water compared to other crops.
* While organic cotton tampons take six months to five years to biodegrade, non-organic tampons take 500–1000 years!
* Disposable pads take 500–800 years to biodegrade.

What else can we use these days?

* Menstrual cups
* Reusable pads
* Period undies
* Menstrual disks

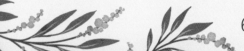

Intention for the week:

MONDAY

SELF-CARE

MEAL PLAN

BODY MOVEMENT

Zᶻᶻ

Today I am grateful for:

TUESDAY

SELF-CARE

MEAL PLAN

BODY MOVEMENT

Zᶻᶻ

Today I am grateful for:

WEDNESDAY

SELF-CARE

MEAL PLAN

BODY MOVEMENT

Zᶻᶻ

Today I am grateful for:

THURSDAY

SELF-CARE

MEAL PLAN

BODY MOVEMENT

Zᶻᶻ

Today I am grateful for:

If you're experiencing PMS, try adding anti-inflammatory foods such as turmeric and estrogen-metabolising foods such as broccoli sprouts to your diet.

FRIDAY

SELF-CARE	MEAL PLAN	BODY MOVEMENT

Zzz

Today I am grateful for:

SATURDAY

SELF-CARE	MEAL PLAN	BODY MOVEMENT

Zzz

Today I am grateful for:

SUNDAY

SELF-CARE	MEAL PLAN	BODY MOVEMENT

Zzz

Today I am grateful for:

Endocrine-disrupting chemicals have been shown to have a negative effect on the hormonal system, affecting everything from skin to fertility. They can be found in many household items such as cleaning and beauty products. Try gradually swapping all these items over to brands that focus on natural ingredients, or even learn how to make your own.

This week, I prioritised my health by . . .

Endometriosis

Over the next few weeks, we're going to learn about a few conditions and phases the body can be in that can affect our cycles and periods. Endometriosis is an inflammatory disease of immune dysfunction that affects at least 1 in 10 people who have or have had a uterus, worldwide. However, an alarming number of people go undiagnosed, with it taking up to 12 years to get a diagnosis.

Endometriosis is the growth of lesions made of a tissue that is very *similar* to our uterine lining, growing outside of the uterus on organs such as the ovaries, fallopian tubes, intestines, bowel and bladder.

Unfortunately, when someone has endometriosis, their immune system responds to the lesions by inflaming and promoting their growth.

The lesions are also affected by the hormones released in the menstrual cycle, which cause the tissue to swell and bleed when you get your period.

However, despite the misconception, endometriosis is not a hormonal condition. Yes, hormones affect it but it's not something that can be healed by balancing hormones. And it isn't caused by hormones being out of balance.

WHAT CAUSES ENDOMETRIOSIS?

What is currently understood is that the immune dysfunction found in endometriosis is caused by a combination of these factors: genetics (if a close relative has endometriosis, you are up to 7 to 10 times more likely to get endometriosis), exposure to toxins that can be found in non-organic plant and animal foods and some rubbers and plastics, leaky gut, nickel allergy, dysfunctional immune system cells, bacterial toxin overgrowth in the pelvis.

WHAT ARE THE SYMPTOMS OF ENDOMETRIOSIS?

If you have the following symptoms, please find a doctor who will investigate further: painful periods, painful sex, pain between periods, pain during urination or bowel movements, pain that makes you vomit or be bed-bound, heavy periods, bleeding from the bladder or bowel, bloating, fatigue, anxiety or depression due to constant pain, difficulty conceiving.

The only way to get a diagnosis is with laparoscopic or keyhole surgery.

HOW TO TREAT ENDOMETRIOSIS?

The top line of defence against endometriosis is having excision surgery to remove the lesions. This is effective in improving pain symptoms and fertility.

However, in about 50% of cases, the lesions grow back within five years, so it's the treatments used after surgery that help achieve long-term health with endo.

Conventional treatment after surgery includes hormonal contraceptives. These can be effective, but they come with their own set of side effects and are not a solution for those who want to start trying to conceive.

There are also natural treatments that can be used to help the body stop producing endometrial lesions and soothe the lesions if they do appear:

* Healing the gut by addressing leaky gut and gut dysbiosis – see Chapter 6.
* Doing a trial of removing inflammatory foods such as gluten and A1 casein dairy, or any food that causes you stomach upset or bloating – see Chapter 8.
* If you are sensitive to nickel jewellery, remove nickel from the diet.
* Taking anti-inflammatory, and immune- and gut-supporting medicines such as:
  * zinc – anti-inflammatory, immune-boosting, can help repair leaky gut, can reduce pain
  * selenium – anti-inflammatory, immune-boosting
  * N-acetyl cysteine – anti-inflammatory, shown to reduce endometrial lesions and reduce the pain of endometriosis
  * turmeric/curcumin – anti-inflammatory and has been found to reduce endometrial lesions
  * berberine – anti-inflammatory, can repair leaky gut and can help reduce the bacterial toxin lipopolysaccharide.

Intention for the week:

MONDAY

SELF-CARE	MEAL PLAN	BODY MOVEMENT

Zᶻ�z

Today I am grateful for:

TUESDAY

SELF-CARE	MEAL PLAN	BODY MOVEMENT

Zᶻz

Today I am grateful for:

WEDNESDAY

SELF-CARE	MEAL PLAN	BODY MOVEMENT

Zᶻz

Today I am grateful for:

THURSDAY

SELF-CARE	MEAL PLAN	BODY MOVEMENT

Zᶻz

Today I am grateful for:

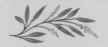

Ashoka is a bark used in Ayurveda to repair the endometrium, regulate estrogen levels, and protect against bacterial and fungal infections such as thrush.

FRIDAY

SELF-CARE	MEAL PLAN	BODY MOVEMENT

Zᶻᶻ

Today I am grateful for:

SATURDAY

SELF-CARE	MEAL PLAN	BODY MOVEMENT

Zᶻᶻ

Today I am grateful for:

SUNDAY

SELF-CARE	MEAL PLAN	BODY MOVEMENT

Zᶻᶻ

Today I am grateful for:

Pelvic inflammatory disease (PID) can occur when bacteria make their way from the vagina to the uterus, fallopian tubes or ovaries. Symptoms include pain and fever.

My favourite moment this week was . . .

Post-birth-control syndrome

and what you can do to avoid it

Full disclaimer – 'post-birth-control syndrome' is not a medically recognised condition. It is, however, treated as a real condition by many complementary practitioners worldwide. And although post-birth-control syndrome is not recognised by the mainstream medical community, the symptoms of post-birth-control syndrome are.

Coming off hormonal birth control isn't necessarily a smooth transition. For some, it comes with many frustrating symptoms. It's when these symptoms persist beyond six months that it may be considered to be post-birth-control syndrome.

SYMPTOMS OF POST-BIRTH-CONTROL SYNDROME

Some of the symptoms include acne, difficulty ovulating, missing periods, depression and anxiety, hair loss, headaches, heavy and painful periods, gut issues and bloating.

Why do these symptoms occur?

It is actually very common for these symptoms to occur when coming off hormonal birth control. Post-birth-control syndrome is only considered once these symptoms persist beyond six months.

Hormonal birth control contains synthetic steroid hormones that suppress the body's ability to create its own hormones. And these synthetic hormones are strong drugs that have side effects.

Transitioning away from these drugs can create a lot of confusion and difficulty inside your body. For example, the steroid hormones in hormonal contraceptives cause your skin to suppress its natural oils. In response to this, your skin creates more oils. When you go off the contraceptive, that suppression is no longer there so all the extra oil your skin has been creating surges to the surface, quite often causing acne.

As another example, the steroid hormones in hormonal contraceptives cause your body to stop producing sex hormones such as estrogen and progesterone. For some, the body does not just bounce back into knowing how to produce those hormones. The endocrine system is delicately balanced and hormonal birth control completely throws that out. It makes sense that the body can take some time to readjust to its natural state, but in the meantime, you may find you don't ovulate or have a regular period.

HOW CAN WE AVOID THESE SYMPTOMS AND POST-BIRTH-CONTROL SYNDROME?

The reality is that you may not be able to avoid it all – but there are things you can do to lessen the effect and put you in the best position possible. As an aside – don't let post-birth-control syndrome scare you into staying on hormonal birth control. There are so many potentially damaging side effects from taking hormonal birth control and so many other ways to handle most symptoms and conditions. Here's what you can do to prepare to come off hormonal birth control (note that you don't have to do these things forever):

* Find a great health practitioner to support you through the transition.
* Consider taking natural acne-preventative medicine such as zinc.
* The pill can create inflammation in the body so reduce inflammation with an anti-inflammatory diet and herbs.
* If you have/had insulin resistance, reduce sugar, balance your carbs with healthy fats and protein, and consider insulin-sensitising supplements such as magnesium.
* The pill depletes the body of many nutrients so consider replenishing magnesium, zinc, selenium, folate, vitamin C, vitamin E and B vitamins through foods and supplements if necessary.
* Support your liver with herbs such as dandelion tea so it can detox the steroid hormones more efficiently.
* Prioritise your gut health with prebiotic and probiotic foods or supplements because the pill can disrupt the gut microbiome.
* Include healthy fats such as nuts, seeds, coconut products and extra virgin olive oil to support your hormone production.

WEEK 15

Intention for the week:

MONDAY

SELF-CARE | MEAL PLAN | BODY MOVEMENT

Z^z_z

Today I am grateful for:

TUESDAY

SELF-CARE | MEAL PLAN | BODY MOVEMENT

Z^z_z

Today I am grateful for:

WEDNESDAY

SELF-CARE | MEAL PLAN | BODY MOVEMENT

Z^z_z

Today I am grateful for:

THURSDAY

SELF-CARE | MEAL PLAN | BODY MOVEMENT

Z^z_z

Today I am grateful for:

Low progesterone levels can result in irregular cycles, difficulty falling pregnant, anxiety . . . the list goes on. Research has shown that a daily dose of 750–1,000 mg of vitamin C can raise progesterone levels.

FRIDAY

SELF-CARE	MEAL PLAN	BODY MOVEMENT
Zzz		

Today I am grateful for:

SATURDAY

SELF-CARE	MEAL PLAN	BODY MOVEMENT
Zzz		

Today I am grateful for:

SUNDAY

SELF-CARE	MEAL PLAN	BODY MOVEMENT
Zzz		

Today I am grateful for:

Drinking spearmint tea has been shown to reduce testosterone levels by up to 30%, greatly slowing the growth of facial hair. It has also been shown to increase important ovulation hormones such as estrogen, lutenising hormone and follicle-stimulating hormone within five days.

Write a thought for someone you miss . . .

Polycystic ovarian syndrome

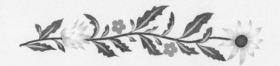

P olycystic ovarian syndrome (PCOS) affects 10–20% of people born with a female hormonal system worldwide. It is the world's leading cause of fertility issues in menstruating people and is a precursor of many serious conditions, including type 2 diabetes, heart disease, endometrial cancer and stroke.

PCOS is an umbrella diagnosis, meaning that it has many varying symptoms, multiple mechanisms driving those symptoms and presents differently for different people.

WHAT CAUSES PCOS?

The cause of PCOS isn't definitive but it can be triggered or driven by exposure to elevated androgens through the mother while in utero, an abnormally rapid pulsatility of gonadotropin-releasing hormone (GnRH), insulin resistance, chronic inflammation, long-term use of hormonal birth control, gut health and stress.

WHAT ARE THE SYMPTOMS OF PCOS?

Symptoms of PCOS include irregular cycles, acne, hirsutism, alopecia, difficulty falling pregnant, weight around the middle, anxiety and depression.

HOW TO GET A DIAGNOSIS

PCOS is currently diagnosed using the Rotterdam Criteria, which states that two of the following three markers need to be present for a diagnosis of PCOS:

1. Anovulation (long or entirely absent cycles)
2. Polycystic ovaries (found using ultrasound)
3. Elevated androgens (either clinical signs such as acne, hirsutism and alopecia, or biochemical signs such as raised testosterone).

However, a new paper released in 2022 disputes the use of the Rotterdam Criteria and shows that PCOS is more accurately defined as a condition of androgen-excess (e.g. high testosterone). It suggests that PCOS should be diagnosed when androgen excess is found and all other causes of androgen excess have been ruled out.

If you suspect you may have PCOS, it's important you get the following hormones and blood-sugar levels tested to determine your drivers and hormonal imbalance: progesterone estrogen, testosterone, DHEA, DHEA-S, DHT, LH, FSH, cortisol, prolactin, cholesterol, fasting insulin, fasting glucose and HbA1C.

LH levels that are elevated in a 2:1 ratio to FSH or higher may indicate your PCOS is driven by dysregulated GnRH. Abnormal fasting insulin, fasting glucose or HbA1C may indicate insulin resistance is driving your PCOS.

Most people with PCOS have higher levels of all androgens. However, for those with adrenal PCOS (i.e. driven by stress) – which is found in about 10% of cases – it is only the DHEA-S androgen that will be elevated.

If you have signs of inflammation such as acne, headaches, joint pain or skin issues, you may also want to test your C-reactive protein (CRP) and erythrocyte sedimentation rate (ESR). If these come back with abnormal levels, inflammation is likely a driver of your PCOS.

HOW TO TREAT PCOS

While there is no definitive cure, effective solutions can be found with herbs and supplements, yoga, massage, meditation, nutrition, lifestyle changes and exercise. Here are some standout medicines to discuss with your practitioner, which can address each driver:

* For GnRH – myo-inositol, cyclic use of oral micronized progesterone
* For insulin resistance – magnesium, chromium, berberine, silymarin, myo-inositol and D-chiro-inositol in a 40:1 ratio
* For inflammation – curcumin, N-acetylcysteine, zinc
* For stress – vitamin B5, ashwagandha, arctic root, L-theanine, cyclic use of oral micronized progesterone, hydrocortisone, liquorice root
* For gut health – see Chapter 6
* For post-pill PCOS, see page 68 on post-birth-control syndrome.

For a list of natural medicines to address each hormonal imbalance, see page 87.

WEEK 16

Intention for the week:

MONDAY

SELF-CARE

Z^z_z

MEAL PLAN

BODY MOVEMENT

Today I am grateful for:

TUESDAY

SELF-CARE

Z^z_z

MEAL PLAN

BODY MOVEMENT

Today I am grateful for:

WEDNESDAY

SELF-CARE

Z^z_z

MEAL PLAN

BODY MOVEMENT

Today I am grateful for:

THURSDAY

SELF-CARE

Z^z_z

MEAL PLAN

BODY MOVEMENT

Today I am grateful for:

A combination of D-chiro inositol and myo-inositol has been well studied and found to be a natural treatment for PCOS that can decrease androgens, regulate the cycle, improve egg quality and ovarian function, and reduce the risk of gestational diabetes.

FRIDAY

SELF-CARE	MEAL PLAN	BODY MOVEMENT

Z^z_z

Today I am grateful for:

SATURDAY

SELF-CARE	MEAL PLAN	BODY MOVEMENT

Z^z_z

Today I am grateful for:

SUNDAY

SELF-CARE	MEAL PLAN	BODY MOVEMENT

Z^z_z

Today I am grateful for:

The combination of liquorice root and peony root has been shown to balance the luteinising hormone to follicle-stimulating hormone (LH:FSH) ratio, support healthy follicle development, increase progesterone levels, reduce elevated androgens, balance blood sugar and reduce inflammation.

Right now, my relationship with myself feels . . .

Menopause

Patriarchy in mind – can every single person reading this (even if you're 15 years old) take a fresh peek at menopause for a sec?

Menopause is almost like a dirty word. So much so that most people have probably skipped past this page. If you're still here reading, yes – we're getting deep and yes – somehow killer whales will be mentioned by the end of it.

If you're like most people, you might have an idea that menopause is like a dreaded end-of-life sentence we inevitably creep towards.

And what seems to be fact is that no matter what, it's going to be uncomfortable. Hot flashes. Sweating. Weight gain. Vaginal dryness. Trouble sleeping. Ugh.

But is this really what's in store? Or is it just the narrative we've been fed?

THE BIOLOGY OF MENOPAUSE

Menopause occurs when the ovaries stop releasing eggs and the production of sex hormones such as estrogen and progesterone decline.

For some people, this change feels intense and the symptoms you've heard of can absolutely be a thing. And that shouldn't be downplayed – funding and research into medical and cultural solutions like paid leave would be great.

For many people, the symptoms are much milder. But regardless of their intensity, these symptoms can be managed with natural medicines and bio-identical hormones. (Talk to a naturopath or functional medicine practitioner!)

Symptom relief is great but the narrative that people should try to avoid or delay menopause completely denies the idea that menopause is actually an incredible transformation. If the narrative around menopause changed to what many postmenopausal people are saying, we'd be hearing a story of freedom – and we might even find it's a transformation to actually look forward to.

THE CULTURE OF MENOPAUSE

Given the inevitability of menopause, we cannot allow it to continue being portrayed in such a negative light. It casts a shadow over our experience of life. Do you think any major area of our life journey should be discussed in such a profoundly negative way?

Does it sound like something the people who actually go through it would have instigated? Hmmm ... we hear the footsteps of the patriarchy ringing in our ears ...

The interesting thing is, once people emerge from the transition of menopause, many are discussing it in an incredibly positive way. Particularly, it provides more sexual freedom and allows them to let go of any menstrual concerns they had. It's been found that people who go into menopause with negative attitudes towards it are more likely to experience a greater number and frequency of symptoms.

Also interesting is the fact that the way menopause is viewed and talked about depends upon culture. In Western society, it is largely medicalised, making menopause feel like a disease state needing treatment.

In Islamic culture and most African cultures, menopause frees people from strict gender roles and people from these societies report fewer symptoms. It is theorised that this is because menopause is seen so positively in their culture.

Menopause is known to only occur in five species on the planet – four types of whales and humans. The life of most female animals comes to an end once their fertility wanes. So why do we (and all those whales) live long lives beyond fertility?

No one knows for sure, but there has been quite a bit of research done into the effect menopause has on orca (killer whale) pods.

Once orcas have gone through menopause, the orca pods, including the males, defer to the postmenopausal whales as their leaders. The older female whales lead their pods, which improves the rate of survival for their offspring.

This progression to leadership can be seen in some human cultures as well. For example, in Aboriginal culture, menopause initiates a gain of status.

What this reflects is the (really, very obvious) view that the wisdom and life experience of postmenopausal people holds worth.

But unfortunately, postmenopausal people in some societies, including Western society, often describe the fact that, despite feeling freer, they also feel like they become invisible after menopause; like their entire existence is pinned upon their ability to procreate and, once that's gone, they're expendable. Do we want to perpetuate this? Or do we want to be a part of a societal shift?

Intention for the week:

MONDAY

SELF-CARE	MEAL PLAN	BODY MOVEMENT

Z^z_z

Today I am grateful for:

TUESDAY

SELF-CARE	MEAL PLAN	BODY MOVEMENT

Z^z_z

Today I am grateful for:

WEDNESDAY

SELF-CARE	MEAL PLAN	BODY MOVEMENT

Z^z_z

Today I am grateful for:

THURSDAY

SELF-CARE	MEAL PLAN	BODY MOVEMENT

Z^z_z

Today I am grateful for:

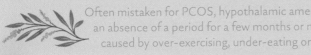
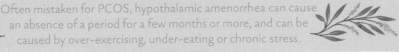

Often mistaken for PCOS, hypothalamic amenorrhea can cause an absence of a period for a few months or more, and can be caused by over-exercising, under-eating or chronic stress.

FRIDAY

SELF-CARE	MEAL PLAN	BODY MOVEMENT

Z^z_z

Today I am grateful for:

SATURDAY

SELF-CARE	MEAL PLAN	BODY MOVEMENT

Z^z_z

Today I am grateful for:

SUNDAY

SELF-CARE	MEAL PLAN	BODY MOVEMENT

Z^z_z

Today I am grateful for:

Perimenopause occurs in the lead-up to entering menopause – it begins 2–10 years prior to your final period. During perimenopause, people can experience symptoms such as hot flashes, irregular cycles, mood swings, vaginal dryness and a decreased sex drive. These symptoms can be managed with the help of supplements such as magnesium.

What is something you can do for yourself today to nurture your health?

Let's reflect ... and talk about the blood

Do you think the info in this chapter has shifted how you will talk about and acknowledge your period socially moving forward?

☐ Definitely

☐ I'm going to be more open about it

☐ Maybe – I like the idea of embracing it all but I'm nervous

☐ Nah, it still feels super private for me and I'm okay with that

After learning about the signs that a cycle is irregular, do you think there is anything you need to discuss with your health practitioner? If so, what are the things you need to discuss?

_____

_____

After reading about tampons and disposable pads, will you keep using them?

☐ Yep! They're my trusty go-to

☐ I don't use them anyway

☐ I'm going to look into using _____ instead!

What's something you learnt about endometriosis that you will remember and can share to help spread awareness?

_____

_____

What's something you learnt about PCOS that you will remember and can share to help spread awareness?

_____

_____

After reading about menopause ... has your perspective changed?

☐ Yes! I'm going to read more about it and try to embrace the transition when it comes

☐ Yes, but it's so far in the future that I'm not going to think about it for a while

☐ I already saw menopause for the magic it is

☐ No – I'm still dreading it!

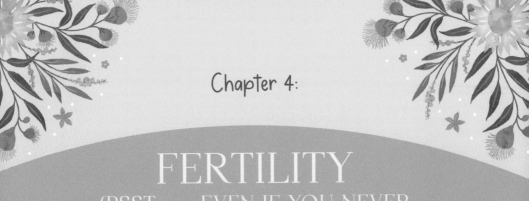

Chapter 4:

FERTILITY
(PSST . . . EVEN IF YOU NEVER WANT TO HAVE A BABY – DON'T SKIP THIS SECTION! YOUR FERTILITY STILL MATTERS!)

Hey, so just wanted to let you know . . . Even if you *never* want to have babies (or having babies is so far in the future that you haven't even thought about your feelings on that yet), your cycle and fertility are still important.

Your fertility isn't just about having a baby. It's a very real and informative insight into your health and it matters.

Plus, this journal is about knowledge building – and your knowledge doesn't just help *you*. Your knowledge about fertility could help a friend, family member or colleague . . . although please, never ever ever ever ever . . . give unsolicited fertility advice to someone trying to conceive. Also, while we're here, never ask anyone if they're pregnant! It's the worst.

In this chapter, we're going to learn about some fundamental factors for reproduction along with some really practical tips for optimising fertility.

You will also find some key information for early pregnancy.

We'd like to issue a **content warning** for this chapter because we will be discussing miscarriage.

If you are trying to conceive, we encourage you to use the cycle tracking chart in the charts section of your journal (see page 233).

To get started though, we want to clear up a misconception about trying to conceive . . .

Natural medicine and making babies

It's important to know there are a tonne of options outside of mainstream Western medicine that can help with fertility. IVF is an option, as is IUI and a range of fertility drugs. And for some people, these options are the perfect fit and lead to beautiful pregnancies and babes. You can talk to a gynaecologist about these options.

But these options aren't the right approach and/or aren't necessary for everyone. They also, usually, don't address the core of what is causing the fertility issue. And the cost of some procedures can make them inaccessible for many.

There are natural options that can be just as effective, if not more so in many scenarios.

But these natural options usually won't be discussed with you by your GP or specialist because, most of the time, natural medicine isn't what they are trained in and so they just are unaware of the options.

This is okay. It doesn't mean the natural options are less valid. It doesn't mean your GP or specialist isn't amazing. It just means there are other options with other experts who can talk to you about them.

Naturopathy, functional medicine, Ayurveda and traditional Chinese medicine offer hundreds of medicines and practices that can be tailored to a treatment program that addresses exactly what is going on in *your* body.

You can even see a natural medicine practitioner alongside your GP or specialist – there are many natural medicines that support and enhance the effects of mainstream Western medicine and fertility procedures.

Natural or pharmaceutical – it's all just medicine. And it's just about finding what *your* body needs.

An important note about progesterone
and early pregnancy

During pregnancy, progesterone is essential for maintaining the uterine lining so the embryo can implant and grow. Without enough progesterone, the baby may miscarry.

Until about 10–12 weeks into pregnancy, the mother's body produces progesterone through the corpus luteum, then after this, the foetus takes over the production of progesterone.

People who are experiencing long or short cycles, have had trouble ovulating, or have hormonal imbalances or trouble conceiving may have low progesterone going into pregnancy. It's integral that during the first trimester, people in these situations have their progesterone levels checked regularly.

If their levels are found to be low, their doctor will prescribe a progesterone supplement to use (it's actually a natural, bio-identical progesterone pessary that is inserted into the vagina each day).

It is important to note that not all general practitioners know about this – it's not their fault, they can't know everything and this seems to be a gap in general knowledge for some practitioners.

So, if you are trying to conceive or you are in your first trimester and you have had hormonal imbalances, irregular cycles or trouble conceiving, advocate for yourself and find a doctor who knows this information and will support you in testing and, if necessary, will help maintain the appropriate levels of progesterone throughout the first trimester. A gynaecologist or OBGYN may be the best person to talk to.

If you never intend to have a baby, this is still good information to have because it is currently largely not known about and it can save the lives and heartache of so many families – so spread the word because it could help one of your friends or family members.

Intention for the week:

MONDAY

SELF-CARE | MEAL PLAN | BODY MOVEMENT

Z^z_z

Today I am grateful for:

TUESDAY

SELF-CARE | MEAL PLAN | BODY MOVEMENT

Z^z_z

Today I am grateful for:

WEDNESDAY

SELF-CARE | MEAL PLAN | BODY MOVEMENT

Z^z_z

Today I am grateful for:

THURSDAY

SELF-CARE | MEAL PLAN | BODY MOVEMENT

Z^z_z

Today I am grateful for:

During IVF, acupuncture has been found to increase follicle numbers, relax uterine muscles and thicken the uterine lining. In one study, acupuncture increased IVF pregnancy rates from 26.3% to 42.5%.

FRIDAY

SELF-CARE	MEAL PLAN	BODY MOVEMENT

Z^z_z

Today I am grateful for:

SATURDAY

SELF-CARE	MEAL PLAN	BODY MOVEMENT

Z^z_z

Today I am grateful for:

SUNDAY

SELF-CARE	MEAL PLAN	BODY MOVEMENT

Z^z_z

Today I am grateful for:

Don't be afraid of seeking help to conceive. It's perfectly natural to help your body be the healthiest it can be and function the best it can. If your arm wasn't working properly, you would go to the doctor. If your teeth hurt when you ate food, you would go to a dentist. You wouldn't feel shame about it. Fertility is just another function of the body – one that is very easy to throw off balance and which commonly needs some adjustment to help it be optimal.

Three things I love about myself are . . .

3 pillars of fertility - pillar 1:
ovulation

When it comes to fertility, there are three areas that can be addressed to optimise your reproductive health. This week, we will cover the first pillar of fertility – ovulation.

As we learnt in Chapter 1, ovulation occurs when an egg is released from one of our ovaries. From there, it is either fertilised by sperm or released along with our uterine lining during our period.

But if your cycle is long or your period is a permanent no-show, it is likely you have a hormonal imbalance that is causing your body to struggle to ovulate. And if you have a regular period but are struggling to fall pregnant, you may actually not be ovulating, even though it seems like you are.

One of the easiest ways to monitor if you are ovulating is by checking your basal body temperature (BBT). If you don't remember the details on this, go back to Chapter 1 where we talk all about BBT.

Just like almost everything with health, the hormonal imbalance that can prevent ovulation is specific to the individual.

A simple blood test of these hormones can help you to understand what hormone/s might be out of balance.

Once you have your test results, you can get a copy and take them to a natural health practitioner such as a naturopath or functional medicine practitioner. They will then tailor a treatment plan that addresses your exact hormone imbalance, while also investigating what might be causing the imbalance to occur.

Under each hormonal imbalance, you will find a list of herbs and supplements that can improve each imbalance, which you can discuss with a natural health practitioner.

High testosterone and other androgens

This can be treated with:

* spearmint tea
* DIM
* berberine
* essential fatty acids
* liquorice and peony root
* myo-inositol and D-chiro-inositolo
* NAC
* selenium
* zinc
* reishi.

High estrogen

This can be treated with:

* vitamin B6
* DIM
* dong quai
* milk thistle
* selenium.

Low estrogen

This can be treated with:

* grapefruit juice
* spearmint tea
* DIM
* dong quai.

An elevated LH:FSH ratio

This can be treated with:

* liquorice and peony root
* apple cider vinegar
* myo-inositol.

High cortisol

This can be treated with:

* ashwagandha
* arctic root
* bacopa
* ginkgo
* cordyceps
* fish oi.

High prolactin

This can be treated with:

* vitamin B6
* vitex (unless LH high)
* removing gluten
* addressing insulin resistance.

Low progesterone

This can be treated with:

* wild yam extract
* vitamin B6
* liquorice and peony root
* bio-identical progesterone
* vitamin C.

With some tests, the above list of supplements in hand, and the help of a good practitioner, you can get to the root cause of what is creating these imbalances, and you can take herbs and supplements to help balance them out.

Other reasons that prevent ovulation include over-exercising, chronic stress and under-eating.

Intention for the week:

MONDAY

SELF-CARE | MEAL PLAN | BODY MOVEMENT

Z^z_z

Today I am grateful for:

TUESDAY

SELF-CARE | MEAL PLAN | BODY MOVEMENT

Z^z_z

Today I am grateful for:

WEDNESDAY

SELF-CARE | MEAL PLAN | BODY MOVEMENT

Z^z_z

Today I am grateful for:

THURSDAY

SELF-CARE | MEAL PLAN | BODY MOVEMENT

Z^z_z

Today I am grateful for:

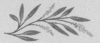

Studies have shown that fertility improves when plant protein is included regularly in our diet. Try integrating lentils, chickpeas and chia seeds into your weekly meals.

FRIDAY

SELF-CARE	MEAL PLAN	BODY MOVEMENT

Z^z_z

Today I am grateful for:

SATURDAY

SELF-CARE	MEAL PLAN	BODY MOVEMENT

Z^z_z

Today I am grateful for:

SUNDAY

SELF-CARE	MEAL PLAN	BODY MOVEMENT

Z^z_z

Today I am grateful for:

Symptoms of having too much estrogen include insomnia, irritability, low libido, bloating, fibroids, PMS, heavy periods, mood swings, anxiety, brain fog, cramps, water retention, sore breasts and migraines. A simple blood test can show you what your estrogen levels are like.

This week, I loved seeing . . .

3 pillars of fertility - pillar 2:

egg quality

Hopefully by now you're feeling super across ovulation – how it happens, what can get in the way and how to optimise it. But what about that little egg you're ovulating? Is it a case of 'it is what it is'? Or can you play a part in it?

There are elements to an egg's quality that you have zero control over. For example, how many chromosomes it has.

There are, however, elements of an egg's quality that we can influence – for example, the powerhouse of the egg cell (and all cells) – the mitochondria.

A healthy egg not only helps the fertilisation and implantation process, but it also affects the viability of a pregnancy.

Although the follicles of our eggs have existed since we were born, the process of maturing a follicle into an egg begins just 90 days or so before the egg is ovulated.

The amazing part of all of this is that during those 90 days, we have the power to impact the health of the egg and that impact can be positive or negative.

There are a number of factors that can damage egg quality in those 90 days, such as stress, hormonal imbalance, sedentary lifestyle, cigarettes, caffeine, alcohol, sugar, soda/soft drink, low-fat diet, processed foods, trans fats, GMO foods and endocrine-disrupting chemicals.

There are also several things you can do to improve egg quality in those 90 days:

Limit the factors that can damage egg quality

These 90 days are such a great opportunity to prioritise your health. Limiting the items that can damage egg quality is great for your overall health, not just your fertility. And in those 90 days, your egg cells are going to have a way better opportunity to thrive and be strong if they are supported.

Eat foods that support egg health

Healthy fats have been found to improve the quality of our eggs. Sources include nuts, seeds, avocado, coconut products, salmon, olive oil, hempseed oil and sunflower sprouts.

Liver contains important nutrients for egg health and for a baby's development.

Beef heart is a fantastic source of CoQ10, which is important for egg health. One way to consume liver and heart (aside from pâté), is to ask your butcher to grind some of it with your beef mince so that it just kind of sneaks in. Good luck to you.

Talk to a natural health practitioner about supplements for egg health

Mitochondria are the part of a cell that can turn the food we eat into the energy the cell can use to function. Mitochondria provide the only source of energy for an egg, and as we age, our mitochondrial function diminishes and can greatly affect egg quality. **CoQ10** can help protect the mitochondria from oxidative stress, allowing it to continue providing energy for the egg. The best form to take is ubiquinol.

Selenium can help to maintain the follicular fluid surrounding the eggs.

Zinc deficiency can negatively affect the early stages of an egg's development, reducing the ability of the egg cells to divide and be fertilised.

NAC helps your body to create glutathione, which is an antioxidant that, like CoQ10, protects the mitochondria.

L-carnitine has been shown to improve ovulation, egg quality and quantity, the health of the endometrium (lining of the womb where the embryo attaches) and the growth of the embryo.

Intention for the week:

MONDAY

SELF-CARE   MEAL PLAN   BODY MOVEMENT

Z^z_z

Today I am grateful for:

TUESDAY

SELF-CARE   MEAL PLAN   BODY MOVEMENT

Z^z_z

Today I am grateful for:

WEDNESDAY

SELF-CARE   MEAL PLAN   BODY MOVEMENT

Z^z_z

Today I am grateful for:

THURSDAY

SELF-CARE   MEAL PLAN   BODY MOVEMENT

Z^z_z

Today I am grateful for:

Being high in healthy fats, fibre, B2, B6, zinc, selenium and magnesium, sunflower seeds can improve fertility and balance hormones. And their phytosterol content helps to reduce cholesterol and supports heart health.

FRIDAY

SELF-CARE	MEAL PLAN	BODY MOVEMENT

Z^z_z

Today I am grateful for:

SATURDAY

SELF-CARE	MEAL PLAN	BODY MOVEMENT

Z^z_z

Today I am grateful for:

SUNDAY

SELF-CARE	MEAL PLAN	BODY MOVEMENT

Z^z_z

Today I am grateful for:

When a fertilised egg attaches itself to the wall of the uterus, it is known as implantation. It happens about 6–12 days after ovulation occurs and, in some people, it causes a small amount of blood to pass. The blood is often a pink or light brown colour.

Right now, I feel like my lifestyle is . . .

3 pillars of fertility - pillar 3:
your reproductive environment

We've covered ovulation and egg quality, but we believe it's the third pillar – reproductive environment – that gets overlooked the most. When we say 'reproductive environment', we're referring to the physical quality of your ovaries, fallopian tubes and uterus.

One of the problems that can occur in the reproductive environment is that it can become 'stagnant' – a term that has a huge focus in Ayurveda and traditional Chinese medicine.

Essentially, a stagnant reproductive system comes down to a lack of blood flow, oxygen and in TCM terms, Qi (energy). Imagine a cold, sluggish, thick, fibrous and clotting environment in your uterus . . . it's not all that inviting or healthy sounding, right?

Symptoms of a stagnant reproductive environment include fibroids; heavy, painful, clotting periods; cysts; slow metabolism; fatigue; cold hands and feet; water retention; and heaviness.

A stagnant reproductive environment can also affect your egg quality – eggs want to be well oxygenated (by blood flow) to implant healthily in the uterus.

If you want to know if stagnation is an issue for you, you can book a session with a TCM or Ayurvedic practitioner.

To improve stagnation, you need to invigorate the area to get your reproductive system energised with plenty of blood flow. Here are some ways you can try:

Heat packs/hot water bottles

This easy DIY method uses heat to help dissolve blockages in the uterus and/or fallopian tubes and prepare the uterine environment for implantation.

It works by promoting blood circulation to wherever the heat is.

Simply place a heat pack or hot-water bottle over your lower abdomen, cover with a towel and lie down to rest, meditate or chill out in front of the TV. Discontinue this practice if you think you may be pregnant.

Fertility massage

This can balance hormones, increase blood circulation in the pelvic area; remove stagnated blood from the reproductive organs; break down fibroids, cysts and uterine scar tissue; stimulate ovulation; ease menstrual pain; and improve egg health. Receiving a fertility massage can be a powerful and enjoyable experience. There are also resources you can purchase online to learn self-fertility-massage techniques.

Red raspberry leaf tea

Drinking red raspberry leaf tea is an easy and delicious way to help circulate fresh blood to the reproductive area, stimulate the ovaries and uterus, and remove congestion. It's a gentle but powerful tea for preparing the uterus for pregnancy. Don't use it if you think you may be pregnant though because it may not be safe.

Yoga

Certain yoga poses can stimulate the reproductive organs and promote blood flow. We list a bunch of these poses on page 102.

Deep breathing

Certain deep breathing practices have been found to increase oxygen levels that our blood can send to every cell in the body. Many practices also promote deep 'belly breathing' that causes your lower abdominal muscles to expand and contract, which attracts blood flow to the lower abdomen. Note that some deep breathing techniques are not recommended if you are pregnant.

Dong quai

This is a powerful root used in TCM to reduce stagnation in the reproductive organs. It may bring on menstruation, balance hormones, reduce inflammation and fatigue, and improve your chances of conceiving. It should not be used during your period, during pregnancy or prior to having surgery, and should only be used with the help of a practitioner.

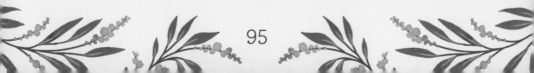

WEEK 21

Intention for the week:

MONDAY

SELF-CARE	MEAL PLAN	BODY MOVEMENT

Z^z_z

Today I am grateful for:

TUESDAY

SELF-CARE	MEAL PLAN	BODY MOVEMENT

Z^z_z

Today I am grateful for:

WEDNESDAY

SELF-CARE	MEAL PLAN	BODY MOVEMENT

Z^z_z

Today I am grateful for:

THURSDAY

SELF-CARE	MEAL PLAN	BODY MOVEMENT

Z^z_z

Today I am grateful for:

Red raspberry leaf tea is great for strengthening and toning the reproductive environment and is also filled with vitamins, antioxidants and iron; can help to prevent blood clots; reduces bloating; and is used by many people in late pregnancy to help prepare for labour.

FRIDAY

SELF-CARE	MEAL PLAN	BODY MOVEMENT
Zᶻᶻ		

Today I am grateful for:

SATURDAY

SELF-CARE	MEAL PLAN	BODY MOVEMENT
Zᶻᶻ		

Today I am grateful for:

SUNDAY

SELF-CARE	MEAL PLAN	BODY MOVEMENT
Zᶻᶻ		

Today I am grateful for:

In TCM, it is believed that the feet should always be kept warm to support the health of your entire body but even more specifically, to support the health of your womb and fertility. It is based on the belief that meridian channels run from your feet through your womb and entire body, so keeping the feet warm keeps your body warm, which is essential for optimal health.

Something I love about my body is . . .

Content warning . . .
(miscarriage)

Miscarriage is such a taboo topic in our society. But if people had more understanding of miscarriage, the people experiencing a loss would be much more supported.

Here are a few insights into miscarriage so you are better able to support a loved one who may go through it and better equipped if you ever face this difficult experience yourself.

THE FACTS

* Miscarriage is the loss of a baby up to 20 weeks' gestation, but most of these losses occur by 12 weeks.
* Miscarriages occur in 10–15% of pregnancies.
* Certain conditions such as PCOS can increase the risk of miscarriage.
* A miscarried baby can pass naturally, which can be painful, or the miscarried baby can be helped out of the uterus by a surgical procedure called a D&C, which requires general anaesthetic.

INSIGHTS FOR HELPING A LOVED ONE WHO HAS MISCARRIED A BABY

* Miscarriage is the loss of a child and often causes complex grief.
* Everyone experiences the grief of a miscarriage differently – never assume how someone is feeling, instead – ask. When someone has lost a baby, it is often all that is on their mind, so you don't need to be afraid of bringing it up – they're probably thinking about it anyway.

* People who miscarry a baby can experience the grief of this for a very long time. However, after the first couple of months, most people around them usually move on and stop checking in with them about it, which can leave them feeling very alone. If you know your loved one can handle talking about it, bringing up the baby is a way to acknowledge that their baby existed and validate their grief.
* Sending messages that require responses in those early days can be too much for someone who has just lost their baby. Instead, sending messages like 'Thinking of you every minute xx' can be a comforting check-in that can be appreciated or responded to.

IF YOU HAVE EXPERIENCED A MISCARRIAGE

* A key consideration for getting through a miscarriage with the best mental health possible is to communicate anything and everything you're feeling with your partner or someone close to you. Experiencing a loss like this has the potential to bring a loving couple even closer together.
* There are many emotions that can be felt when grieving, including anger and guilt. All emotions are valid but recognise if you are feeling these emotions as a distraction from feeling the hardest emotion of all – sadness. Sadness is hard to feel, but it is real and if you feel it in your whole body, you may find that you move through the waves of sadness faster. In saying that, only do what you feel you can manage and ask for support if you need it. Family, friends, therapists, online therapy and counselling lines are all options.
* If you are feeling any negative emotions towards your body, consider the idea that your body is in this with you. This is something that happened to you and your body, not something that your body caused. The aftermath of a miscarriage can be a time for nurturing and nourishing your body and mind, so you can move through this together in a healthy way. Heat packs, self-fertility massage, healing teas like red-raspberry leaf, meditation and yoga are all ways that you can bring love, connection and growth into this devastating time.
* If clicking the on-button on the remote and eating ice cream in your pyjamas is all you can give to life right now, don't worry, that's perfect.

WEEK 22

Intention for the week:

MONDAY

SELF-CARE	MEAL PLAN	BODY MOVEMENT

Z^z_z

Today I am grateful for:

TUESDAY

SELF-CARE	MEAL PLAN	BODY MOVEMENT

Z^z_z

Today I am grateful for:

WEDNESDAY

SELF-CARE	MEAL PLAN	BODY MOVEMENT

Z^z_z

Today I am grateful for:

THURSDAY

SELF-CARE	MEAL PLAN	BODY MOVEMENT

Z^z_z

Today I am grateful for:

'As you breathe in, cherish yourself. As you breathe out, cherish all Beings.' – DALAI LAMA

FRIDAY

SELF-CARE	MEAL PLAN	BODY MOVEMENT

Zᶻᶻ

Today I am grateful for:

SATURDAY

SELF-CARE	MEAL PLAN	BODY MOVEMENT

Zᶻᶻ

Today I am grateful for:

SUNDAY

SELF-CARE	MEAL PLAN	BODY MOVEMENT

Zᶻᶻ

Today I am grateful for:

It might sound strange, but if you want to improve your relationship with your body, you could start by actually imagining you're in a relationship with it. When it says it's full or hungry, respond to that message. When it says it's tired, sleep. And imagine that it can hear everything you say and think – would you want someone you're in a relationship with to hear you say negative things about them? Try treating your body with love, respect, gratitude and compassion – like you would any relationship.

Something healthy that makes me feel great is . . .

Yoga poses for fertility and cycle health

Yoga has been studied and shown to have incredible effects on our fertility and cycle health, including regulating cycle length, balancing hormones and even supporting sperm production. It is also fantastic for circulating blood around the body including to the reproductive organs, which can energise, refresh and strengthen those important organs that are necessary for fertility and cycle health.

Practising one or a combination of these poses regularly is a practical DIY way to support your cycle and fertility.

Legs up the wall pose

Can regulate hormones, bring blood flow to the reproductive organs and energise the pelvic area. Practise this pose with a cushion underneath your hips.

Butterfly pose

Can open and relax your pelvic area.

Mill churning pose

Can normalise the function of your reproductive organs, balance your hormones and help you lose weight.

Child's pose

Can soothe your central nervous system and relieve menstrual cramps and symptoms of PMS.

Bharadvaja's twist

Can soothe your nervous system, balance blood pressure and regulate menstruation.

Cobra pose

Can stimulate ovarian function, improve digestion and reduce stress.

Lotus pose

Can help stretch the pelvic area, balance your hormones, reduce menstrual discomfort and ease childbirth.

Cat–cow pose

Can stimulate your reproductive organs and enhance the function of your central nervous system.

Superman pose

Can tone your stomach and increase blood flow to your reproductive organs.

Bow pose

Can stimulate your reproductive organs, relieve menstrual discomfort and normalise your cycle.

Wide-legged forward bend

Can increase blood circulation to the ovaries.

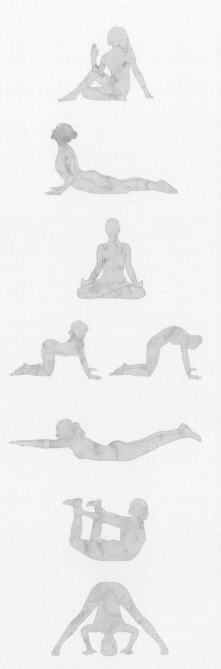

Intention for the week:

MONDAY

SELF-CARE | MEAL PLAN | BODY MOVEMENT

Z^z_z

Today I am grateful for:

TUESDAY

SELF-CARE | MEAL PLAN | BODY MOVEMENT

Z^z_z

Today I am grateful for:

WEDNESDAY

SELF-CARE | MEAL PLAN | BODY MOVEMENT

Z^z_z

Today I am grateful for:

THURSDAY

SELF-CARE | MEAL PLAN | BODY MOVEMENT

Z^z_z

Today I am grateful for:

Although caesarean deliveries occur in a more sterile environment, they are still sacred and can feel just as exciting and special as a vaginal delivery. You can talk to your doctor about ways to make the delivery feel more tailored to you, e.g. music, a quiet room, delayed cord clamping and skin-to-skin.

FRIDAY

SELF-CARE	MEAL PLAN	BODY MOVEMENT
Z^z_z		

Today I am grateful for:

SATURDAY

SELF-CARE	MEAL PLAN	BODY MOVEMENT
Z^z_z		

Today I am grateful for:

SUNDAY

SELF-CARE	MEAL PLAN	BODY MOVEMENT
Z^z_z		

Today I am grateful for:

The World Health Organization recommends breastfeeding 'up to two years and beyond', with natural weaning often occurring between four and five years of age. The judgement of breastfeeding beyond infancy is medically unfounded and socially born in the 1800s by the upper class who decided breastfeeding was only done by 'uneducated' people who couldn't afford formula. In saying that, the health and happiness of the mother is paramount. If breastfeeding isn't conducive to that, there are fantastic formulas available.

This week, I feel proud of myself for . . .

Let's reflect . . .

Are there any practical steps you plan to take to support your fertility?

_____

_____

If you are trying to conceive, is there anything you've learnt in this chapter that you would like to bring up with your health practitioner?

_____

_____

Do you know if you are ovulating?

☐ Yes, I'm definitely ovulating

☐ I'm really not sure and I'm going to talk to my doctor about it

☐ I'm not ovulating because I'm on hormonal birth control

☐ I'm not ovulating and I'm going to get some hormone testing done to find out why

Are there any herbs or supplements for hormonal imbalance that you want to talk to your health practitioner about?

_____

_____

Are you going to take any steps to support your egg health?

_____

_____

Will you be taking any steps to support your reproductive environment?

_____

_____

Will you be incorporating any yoga poses for your cycle and fertility health?

_____

_____

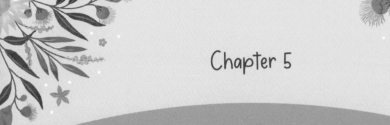

Chapter 5

MENTAL HEALTH ... AKA HEALTH

Your mind and your body are one and the same. And the health of your mind can influence the health of the rest of your body (and vice versa).

In this chapter, we will look at the biological (internal body) systems that underpin our mental health, the conditions that can affect us and the many ways we can seek help and improve our mental health.

What we hope is that, by the end of this chapter, you will feel how important it is to prioritise your mental health, how connected your mental health is to your physical health, and how acceptable and normal it is to receive support from mental health practitioners.

If anything in this chapter resonates, triggers anything or even just makes you wonder, get in touch with your health professional as a matter of priority, call a helpline or sign up to an online therapy service.

And please note a content warning on this chapter – we do discuss mental health issues and trauma.

Mental health

it's an emotions thing, right?

With roughly 10% of the world experiencing mental health issues (make that 20–30% in the Western world), it's safe to say that mental health is super important *and* needs addressing.

Women are also more likely to experience mental health issues with approximately 1 in 3 Australian women experiencing anxiety in their lifetime.

WHAT'S CAUSING MENTAL HEALTH ISSUES?

Most of us can understand that distressing, traumatic and emotional experiences can lead to mental health issues, but what many people don't know is that there are other factors that can affect our mental health.

Interestingly too, the scientific world can't even agree upon the mechanisms of mental health. Is it a physical disease of the brain? Or is it emotionally or spiritually driven . . .

What is agreed is that the scientific understanding of mental health is far behind that of other areas of the body, and many developments in our understanding lie ahead of us. Which is exciting for the future.

In saying that, there are three areas at play when it comes to mental health. Below, we have listed those areas and the elements that can affect us.

Our external world

* Difficult or abusive relationships
* Work pressures, struggles and satisfaction
* Balance of work and other activities
* Financial pressures
* Lack of or too strenuous exercise
* Not enough exposure to nature or natural light
* Inadequate sleep
* Dysregulated breathing patterns
* Our response to change

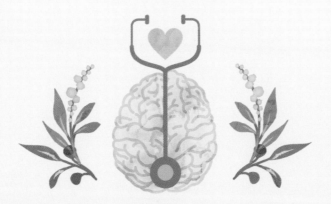

Our internal world

* Negative thoughts and beliefs
* Past or present trauma
* Chronic stress
* Perceived lack of purpose
* Nervous system dysregulation
* Addiction (although this is listed as a cause, addiction is a symptom of trauma/pain. It does feed mental health issues but only because it was first fed by emotional issues)

Our biological body

* Gut health
* Hormonal imbalance
* Genetics
* Inflammation
* Nutrient deficiencies
* Toxins
* Imbalanced neurotransmitters such as serotonin and dopamine (our 'happy hormones')
* Issues with mitochondria (the energy for each cell of the body)

Yep, each of these things can drive mental health issues. This means that mental health isn't just caused by difficult experiences or emotionally driven responses but also by physical factors, like the health of our gut and how much sun we're getting.

When we do have a mental health issue, it's important to consider all of these factors and address any we think might need changing. This chapter provides insights into how and why some of these factors come about, and what you can do about them.

Intention for the week:

MONDAY

SELF-CARE	MEAL PLAN	BODY MOVEMENT

Z^z_z

Today I am grateful for:

TUESDAY

SELF-CARE	MEAL PLAN	BODY MOVEMENT

Z^z_z

Today I am grateful for:

WEDNESDAY

SELF-CARE	MEAL PLAN	BODY MOVEMENT

Z^z_z

Today I am grateful for:

THURSDAY

SELF-CARE	MEAL PLAN	BODY MOVEMENT

Z^z_z

Today I am grateful for:

Adaptogens such as ashwagandha, maca and golden root are a class of herbs that are neither stimulating or sedating, but bring hormones, stress levels and the body into a state of balance known as homeostasis. Talk to a natural health practitioner about adaptogens that may suit your body.

FRIDAY

SELF-CARE	MEAL PLAN	BODY MOVEMENT

Z^zz

Today I am grateful for:

SATURDAY

SELF-CARE	MEAL PLAN	BODY MOVEMENT

Z^zz

Today I am grateful for:

SUNDAY

SELF-CARE	MEAL PLAN	BODY MOVEMENT

Z^zz

Today I am grateful for:

In Chinese medicine, it is believed that every biological and energetic system in the body is reflected in the ears. When you massage your ears, you are stimulating the energy points and meridians that connect to the whole body, clearing blockages and helping to heal a huge range of physical and mental health issues. It also stimulates nerve endings, which release endorphins. Ear massage feels great and can be done as often as you like; however, it may need to be avoided if pregnant.

This week, I prioritised my health by . . .

The reality of stress

Arguably, one of the biggest factors that can drive mental and chronic health issues is stress. And we know everyone says 'stress can make you sick' . . . but like, for real. Stress can make you sick.

The main reason stress has such a huge impact is cortisol.

Cortisol is a hormone released by your adrenal glands in response to stress. It helps you handle stress and survive dangerous situations.

Unfortunately, our stressful lifestyles can cause us to release cortisol too frequently.

Every time we feel intense stress, our body interprets that stress as a physical threat, activating our fight or flight response and releasing cortisol, which increases our blood-sugar levels so we have more energy, increases our blood pressure to pump more blood to our limbs, increases our breath rate to increase oxygen, impairs our immune system so our body can focus on the task at hand rather than healing existing conditions, and slows down our digestion. This is all so our body can focus on surviving the 'situation' we are in.

Our body is thinking the situation is life or death. It's picturing a tiger or a fast-moving car. But the reality is, we're usually sitting at a desk, lying in bed or waiting in traffic. This false alarm can be truly damaging.

SYMPTOMS OF HIGH CORTISOL

Symptoms of high cortisol include acne, facial hair, irregular menstrual cycles, weight gain (particularly around the abdomen and face), digestive issues, difficulty sleeping, fatigue, unhealthy food cravings, low libido, mood swings, irritability, poor concentration, poor memory, anxiety and depression.

HOW DO HIGH LEVELS OF CORTISOL AFFECT THE BODY?

Our hormones

High levels of cortisol can cause an increase in androgens and insulin, and difficulty responding to other hormones such as progesterone. This can lead to issues with insulin resistance, fertility, thyroid function and metabolism.

Our neurotransmitters

Chronic stress and cortisol can cause a decrease in serotonin and GABA – two neurotransmitters (happy hormones) that are crucial for sleep, digestion, weight, sense of wellbeing and mental health.

Our nervous system

The nervous system is the body's communication system – it takes in all the internal and external information and sends it around your body, telling your body what to do with the information. It is also the home of our fight or flight response. When we feel chronic stress and continually release cortisol, the fight or flight response can become so constant it can struggle to switch off and our nervous system can become dysregulated – affecting how we feel, think, react and behave. A dysregulated nervous system can cause anxiety, depression, PTSD, OCD, ADHD, insomnia and addiction. It can make relationships very difficult because it can cause outbursts, irrational anger, overreactions and generally dysfunctional behaviour. And it can also cause physical symptoms such as cravings, insatiable hunger, fatigue, constipation, bloating, cramps, sore boobs, difficulty ovulating, low immunity, and body aches and pains.

The good news is we can turn all of this around!

Manage your stress and cortisol levels by getting adequate sleep; doing regular, nurturing exercise; practising meditation, mindfulness and relaxation; and talking to a health practitioner about herbs and supplements such as ashwaghanda (can reduce cortisol by 30%), arctic root (can reduce cortisol, increase resilience to stress, reduce depression by 50% and increase our happy hormones) and L-Theanine (can reduce stress and cortisol levels for up to three hours).

Intention for the week:

MONDAY

SELF-CARE	MEAL PLAN	BODY MOVEMENT

Z^z_z

Today I am grateful for:

TUESDAY

SELF-CARE	MEAL PLAN	BODY MOVEMENT

Z^z_z

Today I am grateful for:

WEDNESDAY

SELF-CARE	MEAL PLAN	BODY MOVEMENT

Z^z_z

Today I am grateful for:

THURSDAY

SELF-CARE	MEAL PLAN	BODY MOVEMENT

Z^z_z

Today I am grateful for:

The vagus nerve runs from the brain through the throat to the digestive system. When the vagus nerve senses long, slow breaths passing over it in the throat, it tells the brain that everything is okay and switches your body from fight or flight to rest and digest. This can be powerful in stressful situations.

FRIDAY

SELF-CARE	MEAL PLAN	BODY MOVEMENT

Zᶻᶻ

Today I am grateful for:

SATURDAY

SELF-CARE	MEAL PLAN	BODY MOVEMENT

Zᶻᶻ

Today I am grateful for:

SUNDAY

SELF-CARE	MEAL PLAN	BODY MOVEMENT

Zᶻᶻ

Today I am grateful for:

A dysregulated nervous system can be caused by trauma, chronic stress, addictive substances, big life changes, grief, mould, heavy metals and chronic infections. To heal it, work with a functional medicine doctor and a mental health practitioner who specialises in mind-body therapies, introduce regular relaxation practices to your day, assess if your hormonal system and gut health need addressing, and ensure you're getting proper sleep and regular exercise.

My favourite moment this week was . . .

Types of depression

Many people have a preconceived notion of what depression is, how it looks and how it might feel. But depression is complex. It can show up in different ways and because it is so misunderstood, sometimes it can go unnoticed.

Below are the types of depressive disorders that can be experienced and some of their distinguishing characteristics.

Remember – if any of this resonates, triggers anything or even just makes you wonder, get in touch with your health professional as a matter of priority, call a helpline or sign up to an online therapy service.

Major depression

* It's sometimes called major depressive disorder, clinical depression, unipolar depression or 'depression'.
* Characterised by low mood and a loss of interest or pleasure.
* Symptoms are experienced most days and last for at least two weeks.
* Symptoms affect and interfere with all aspects of a person's life.
* Major depression can be described as mild, moderate or severe.
* Major depression has the following sub-categories:
    - **Melancholia** – severe depression, move slower, loss of pleasure
    - **Psychotic depression** – hallucinations, delusions, paranoia
    - **Antenatal and postnatal depression** – can occur during pregnancy or in the first year after giving birth, crying regularly for more than two weeks, unwanted thoughts, struggle to connect with the baby, guilt, hopelessness, feeling panicky, loss of confidence. Can be triggered by dramatic drop in estrogen and progesterone after delivery.

Bi-polar disorder

* Previously known as 'manic depression'
* Periods of depression, mania and normal mood in between
* Typically cycle through these episodes twice per year.
* Manic periods are characterised by high energy, racing thoughts, needing little sleep, fast talking, difficulty focusing, irritability.
* Manic periods can include hallucinations and delusions.
* 80% of cases are inherited genetically.
* Can be triggered by stressful events and also by the onset of spring, due to the increase in sunlight hours affecting the pineal gland.
  * **Bi-polar disorder has the following sub-categories** – bi-polar 1, bi-polar 2, cyclothymic disorder and a category called 'other types'

Dysthymic disorder

* Mild depression
* Lasts at least two years

Seasonal affective disorder (SAD)

* Depression or mania caused by seasonal changes
* Most common form of SAD is depression beginning in winter and ending at the onset of spring.
* Diagnosed when someone experiences this pattern for two years or more.
* Symptoms include a lack of energy, sleeping a lot, overeating.

Atypical depression

* The same as major depression; however, symptoms relieved and mood improved when positive events happen.

Adjustment disorder with depressed mood

* Looks like major depression, but is triggered by a specific event such as the death of a loved one
* Extremity and length of the depressive mood out of proportion with the event.

Intention for the week:

MONDAY

SELF-CARE	MEAL PLAN	BODY MOVEMENT

Z^z_z

Today I am grateful for:

TUESDAY

SELF-CARE	MEAL PLAN	BODY MOVEMENT

Z^z_z

Today I am grateful for:

WEDNESDAY

SELF-CARE	MEAL PLAN	BODY MOVEMENT

Z^z_z

Today I am grateful for:

THURSDAY

SELF-CARE	MEAL PLAN	BODY MOVEMENT

Z^z_z

Today I am grateful for:

Nothing is impossible. The word itself says 'I'm possible'! - AUDREY HEPBURN

	SELF-CARE	MEAL PLAN	BODY MOVEMENT
FRIDAY	Z^z_z		

Today I am grateful for:

	SELF-CARE	MEAL PLAN	BODY MOVEMENT
SATURDAY	Z^z_z		

Today I am grateful for:

	SELF-CARE	MEAL PLAN	BODY MOVEMENT
SUNDAY	Z^z_z		

Today I am grateful for:

SAM-e is a compound found naturally in the body that can increase dopamine and serotonin levels when taken by people experiencing depression.

Check in! How are your intentions for the year going? Are there things you can do to help progress them? Are your intentions still meaningful to you or do they need an update?

The signs and symptoms of anxiety

Anxiety can present in a number of ways and to varying degrees, and it's normal for people to feel a little anxiety from time to time. What is for sure is that if you are suffering from these symptoms regularly or if they are affecting any part of your life, you should seek help.

Seeking help for your mental health is total self-care! It's a dedication to your health and what's not to love about prioritising yourself and paying attention to your wonderful mind.

THE SIGNS

Psychological

* Excessive fear
* Worry
* Catastrophising
* Obsessive thinking
* Dread
* Nervousness
* Phobias
* Difficulty concentrating

Physical

* Racing heart
* Tight chest
* Panic attacks
* Hot and cold flushes
* Feeling tense and on edge
* Rapid breathing
* Trouble sleeping
* Feeling weak or tired

Behavioural

* Avoiding certain situations because of feeling anxious
* Inability to speak
* Procrastination
* Difficulty making decisions
* Social withdrawal

Ways to address anxiety and depression

There are *so many* ways to address anxiety and depression. All is not lost! You don't necessarily need to feel this way forever. And if you've tried something in the past and it hasn't helped, have a look at all the options below, pick the one that feels the most appealing, find a practitioner and go for it.

Therapy

* Cognitive behavioural therapy
* Eye movement desensitisation and reprocessing (EMDR) therapy
* Dialectical behavioural therapy
* Psychodynamic therapy
* Humanistic therapy
* Psychoanalytic therapy

Medicine

* Medication from a GP or psychiatrist including SSRIs, SNRIs, benzodiazepines and tricyclic antidepressants.
* Herbs and supplements from a natural health practitioner such as ashwaghanda, St John's wort, arctic root, SAM-e, phenethylamine (PEA), L-theanine, prebiotics and probiotics

Lifestyle practices

* Slow, deep breathing
* Exercise
* Adequate sleep
* Meditation, mindfulness and relaxation
* Daily gratitude
* Listening to music
* Yoga
* Being in nature
* Getting natural light

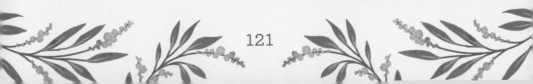

Intention for the week:

MONDAY

SELF-CARE	MEAL PLAN	BODY MOVEMENT

Z$_z^z$

Today I am grateful for:

TUESDAY

SELF-CARE	MEAL PLAN	BODY MOVEMENT

Z$_z^z$

Today I am grateful for:

WEDNESDAY

SELF-CARE	MEAL PLAN	BODY MOVEMENT

Z$_z^z$

Today I am grateful for:

THURSDAY

SELF-CARE	MEAL PLAN	BODY MOVEMENT

Z$_z^z$

Today I am grateful for:

It can be important to reflect on how your mood has been. If it has been low on more days than you would like, perhaps talk to a friend or a counsellor.

FRIDAY

SELF-CARE	MEAL PLAN	BODY MOVEMENT

Zzz

Today I am grateful for:

SATURDAY

SELF-CARE	MEAL PLAN	BODY MOVEMENT

Zzz

Today I am grateful for:

SUNDAY

SELF-CARE	MEAL PLAN	BODY MOVEMENT

Zzz

Today I am grateful for:

Our neurotransmitters (happy hormones such as dopamine and serotonin) can be reduced by things like nutrient deficiencies, eating too few carbs, hormonal imbalances, stress, poor sleep and gut issues. Western medicine uses SSRI anti-depressant medication to increase serotonin levels. Natural medicine practitioners may prescribe amino acids such as PEA and L-theanine to increase neurotransmitters.

Make a list of the precious people in your life who support you. If you think the list is too short, perhaps try reaching out to someone; they may need you as much as you need them.

PMS or PMDD?

M ost of us have heard of PMS, AKA premenstrual syndrome. But many of us haven't heard of its super-intense cousin, premenstrual dysphoric disorder (PMDD).

PMDD is considered an endocrine (hormonal) disorder and has a whole range of physical symptoms. But we have included it in this chapter because of the heavy toll it can take on a person's mental health. And because it can be misdiagnosed for other mental health conditions.

PMS and PMDD have their similarities, which is why PMDD is often missed in the roughly 8% of people who have it. But how they differ is in their intensity, frequency and duration.

Check out the differences between PMS and PMDD, which follow, and take note of how you feel in the lead-up to your period.

PMS

* Symptoms appear 5–7 days before period
* Up to five symptoms
* Experienced on some cycles
* Uncomfortable but usually can function

PMDD

* Symptoms appear up to 14 days before period
* Five or more symptoms
* Experienced most cycles
* Severe, often debilitating and can be damaging to relationships, work and study.

PMS symptoms

* Acne
* Breast tenderness
* Irritability
* Anxiety and depression
* Insomnia
* Bloating
* Cramping
* Headaches
* Cravings
* Mood swings
* Crying
* Poor concentration
* Low energy
* Constipation or diarrhea
* Water retention

PMDD symptoms

* PMS symptoms (see list, left)
* Rage
* Joint pain
* Extreme fatigue
* Suicidal thoughts
* Severe depressive feelings of Hopelessness lack of interest and sadness
* Hot flashes
* Muscle pain and spasms
* Lack of control
* Confusion
* Vision changes
* Allergies
* Skin issues like itching and cold sores
* Fainting
* Heart palpitations

Intention for the week:

MONDAY

SELF-CARE	MEAL PLAN	BODY MOVEMENT
Z^z_z		

Today I am grateful for:

TUESDAY

SELF-CARE	MEAL PLAN	BODY MOVEMENT
Z^z_z		

Today I am grateful for:

WEDNESDAY

SELF-CARE	MEAL PLAN	BODY MOVEMENT
Z^z_z		

Today I am grateful for:

THURSDAY

SELF-CARE	MEAL PLAN	BODY MOVEMENT
Z^z_z		

Today I am grateful for:

The level of stress caused by an event, experience or worry is subjective. It depends on your reaction to the stressor. If you become stressed easily, stress management and resilience techniques like mindfulness, yoga and deep breathing may benefit you.

FRIDAY

SELF-CARE	MEAL PLAN	BODY MOVEMENT
Zzz		

Today I am grateful for:

SATURDAY

SELF-CARE	MEAL PLAN	BODY MOVEMENT
Zzz		

Today I am grateful for:

SUNDAY

SELF-CARE	MEAL PLAN	BODY MOVEMENT
Zzz		

Today I am grateful for:

The hypothalamic-pituitary-adrenal (HPA) axis is activated in response to stress, producing the hormone cortisol. The HPA axis isn't just activated by current stress but by thoughts or triggers of past stressors. When this happens, the cortisol response is activated for a longer period, which can be more damaging. Our thoughts are powerful – increasing our resilience to stress is an important part of maintaining hormonal balance and good mental health.

Right now, my relationship with myself feels . . .

Trauma and EMDR

Usually, when people think of 'trauma', they imagine traumatic, dramatic events. And yes, traumatic events are a thing and many people have post-traumatic stress disorder (PTSD) because of them.

But trauma can also come about from smaller, everyday experiences. And childhood trauma can stem from *so many* situations – from the obvious experiences of neglect to the more nuanced experiences of an unstable environment.

Recommended ways to treat trauma include cognitive processing therapy, trauma-focused cognitive behavioural therapy, cognitive therapy and prolonged exposure.

One recommended option we want to focus on is EMDR – eye movement desensitisation and reprocessing. And despite its *long* name, one of its benefits is its potentially *short* timeframe for seeing results.

WHAT ON EARTH IS EMDR?

EMDR is a psychological treatment developed about 30 years ago. It has primarily been used to treat trauma and the reason we want to highlight it is because it has become the *most* researched therapeutic approach for PTSD. It is also now being used more widely to treat an array of issues including anxiety, depression, eating disorders and phobias, with research showing incredibly good results.

EMDR therapists use a rapid eye movement technique to help patients heal from the symptoms and emotional distress that result from difficult life experiences and memories.

EMDR is a therapy with standardised procedures, meaning that practitioners follow a set process to perform EMDR. It is an eight-phase treatment process that begins with the practitioner learning about the patient – their symptoms, support network and self-regulation abilities – and ensuring if the patient's scenario would suit EMDR.

The EMDR therapist then works through difficult life events, one memory at a time. EMDR can help patients process the memory more fully and quite quickly move their reaction to that memory from a negative place to one of acceptance and even empowerment.

It should be noted, however, that this can be an intense experience. To do EMDR you will need to be actively thinking about these memories and reflecting on your reaction to them, while using your eyes to follow the therapist's hand back and forth. Also note, this is not a form of hypnotherapy; it has to do with the rapid eye movement experienced in REM sleep and the effect that it can have on the brain's ability to process.

For someone suffering with a single experience of PTSD, it may only be one or two memories that need to be worked through. For others suffering with multiple difficult life events and memories, the treatment process will be applied to each memory, one at a time.

The amazing thing is that these memories can often be worked through incredibly quickly, with multiple memories sometimes being processed in a single 60-minute session.

Studies have shown that 84–90% of people suffering from single-event PTSD have been healed in just three 90-minute sessions. One study showed that 100% of single-trauma victims and 77% of multiple trauma victims were no longer diagnosed with PTSD after just six 50-minute sessions.

EMDR isn't for everyone. But, dark leafy greens aside, nothing is for everyone. What is for sure is that if you have experienced trauma, have been diagnosed with PTSD, are considering therapy or are looking to change your current therapy plan, EMDR is an effective and available option – one that many people haven't heard about but is offered all around the world.

Intention for the week:

MONDAY

SELF-CARE | MEAL PLAN | BODY MOVEMENT

Z^z_z

Today I am grateful for:

TUESDAY

SELF-CARE | MEAL PLAN | BODY MOVEMENT

Z^z_z

Today I am grateful for:

WEDNESDAY

SELF-CARE | MEAL PLAN | BODY MOVEMENT

Z^z_z

Today I am grateful for:

THURSDAY

SELF-CARE | MEAL PLAN | BODY MOVEMENT

Z^z_z

Today I am grateful for:

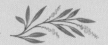

FRIDAY

SELF-CARE	MEAL PLAN	BODY MOVEMENT
Z^z_z		

Today I am grateful for:

SATURDAY

SELF-CARE	MEAL PLAN	BODY MOVEMENT
Z^z_z		

Today I am grateful for:

SUNDAY

SELF-CARE	MEAL PLAN	BODY MOVEMENT
Z^z_z		

Today I am grateful for:

Meditation, mindfulness and relaxation are similar but distinct types of practice. Relaxation is consciously letting go of tension in the physical body, relaxing the mind. Mindfulness is being aware in the moment, releasing worries, bringing ease and comfort. Meditation is withdrawing your senses from the external and bringing your awareness inside, creating the opportunity for deep rejuvenation and bliss.

What is something you can do for yourself today to nurture your health?

Yoga poses for mental health

Yoga is no joke! Studies have found it can significantly reduce depression, anxiety and stress, and importantly, it can also improve the way we respond to stressful situations.

Check out these poses that can specifically help with anxiety, depression, stress and mood.

Tree pose

Can increase serotonin (a happy hormone), help you focus inwards and quiet racing thoughts.

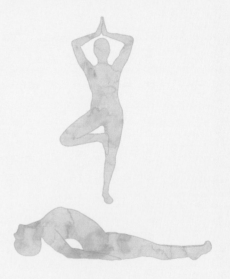

Fish pose

Can help you to relieve tightness in your chest, release pent-up emotions and feel calmer.

Bridge pose

Can improve symptoms of stress, anxiety and depression.

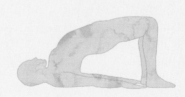

Child's pose

Can calm the nervous system, easing stress, anxiety and fatigue.

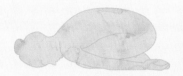

Seated forward bend

Can calm the mind and relieve symptoms of anxiety and stress.

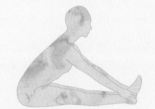

Legs up the wall pose

Can completely relax your mind and body. Practise this pose with a cushion underneath your hips.

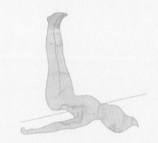

Downward-facing dog pose

Can increase blood circulation to the brain, improving mood.

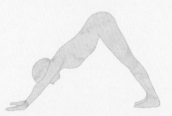

Dolphin pose

Can help with insomnia and mild symptoms of depression.

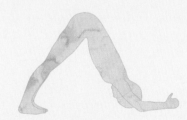

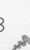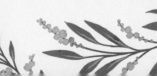

Intention for the week:

MONDAY

SELF-CARE

MEAL PLAN

BODY MOVEMENT

Z^z_z

Today I am grateful for:

TUESDAY

SELF-CARE

MEAL PLAN

BODY MOVEMENT

Z^z_z

Today I am grateful for:

WEDNESDAY

SELF-CARE

MEAL PLAN

BODY MOVEMENT

Z^z_z

Today I am grateful for:

THURSDAY

SELF-CARE

MEAL PLAN

BODY MOVEMENT

Z^z_z

Today I am grateful for:

FRIDAY

SELF-CARE	MEAL PLAN	BODY MOVEMENT
Zzᶻ		

Today I am grateful for:

SATURDAY

SELF-CARE	MEAL PLAN	BODY MOVEMENT
Zzᶻ		

Today I am grateful for:

SUNDAY

SELF-CARE	MEAL PLAN	BODY MOVEMENT
Zzᶻ		

Today I am grateful for:

It has been found that girls and women are consistently underdiagnosed with ADHD. This is because girls and women tend to have fewer external symptoms, and because doctors have historically thought of ADHD as a male condition. Symptoms of ADHD in women such as chattiness, spaciness and forgetfulness are often explained away as personality traits.

Three things I love about myself are . . .

How are you feeling?

Do you think any of the 'external world', 'internal world' or 'biological body' factors have been affecting your mental health? What are they and how long do you think they've been an issue for?

_____

_____

Do you think stress and cortisol are having an impact on your life?

☐ 100% – I'm going to do something about it

☐ 100% – but I feel there isn't much I can change so I need to discuss it with a health practitioner

☐ I have stress in my life but I think I'm managing it really well

☐ I couldn't be more relaxed

Do you have any symptoms of high cortisol?

_____

_____

Do you think your nervous system could be dysregulated?

☐ 100% – I am working/need to work on this with a health practitioner

☐ I'm not sure and will discuss it with my health practitioner

☐ No way, I feel healthy and balanced

If you've found that stress, cortisol or any of the other causes of mental health issues are affecting you, what plans can you make to do something about addressing them?

_____

_____

Are there any mental health treatment methods you now know about that you would like to explore with your health practitioner?

_____

_____

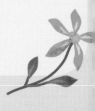

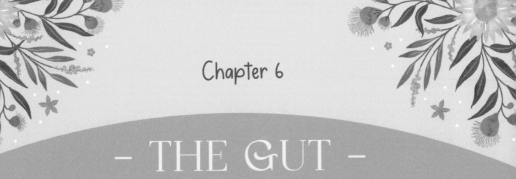

Chapter 6

– THE GUT –
WHO EVEN KNEW IT WAS THE EPICENTRE OF HEALTH?

The gut encompasses all the organs that food passes through, from the mouth to the anus, but what is incredible about the gut is that it isn't just food that you will find inside it.

Living their lives throughout the gut are literally *trillions* of microscopic organisms – mainly fungus, pathogens and bacteria.

We are in a symbiotic relationship with these little guys and most of us don't even know it.

As a collective, these organisms are called the 'gut microbiome' and they have evolved to live inside the human body. Your body is their entire word. Their home. And just like the earth affects our health, we affect the health of these trillions of organisms. And just like our existence affects the health of the planet, these organisms affect us.

A large portion of your microbiome is made up of good and bad bacteria. An imbalance of these bacteria can lead to many health issues for both our mind and physical body.

But your microbiome isn't the only element of your gut that affects your health.

Throughout this chapter, we will look at the many ways our gut affects our health and what we can do about it.

We will also look at the functions of the gut and the organs that support it.

There is growing evidence showing that the gut is central to our health, and that healing our gut and prioritising its health could be the missing piece of the puzzle for many people who are suffering.

Bacteria

The friends we didn't know we had

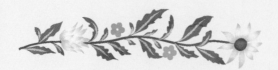

Our microbiome does part of the work of the human body. As in, some of the things you think 'you' are responsible for are actually being done by the good bacteria in your gut. For example, good bacteria help you with the breakdown and absorption of food.

They also protect us from dangerous pathogens and help to create neurotransmitters such as serotonin (happy hormone), dopamine (pleasure hormone), melatonin (sleep hormone) and acetylcholine (attention, learning and memory hormone). You read that right – hormones that *you* need for things like mental health, are actually being created by foreign entities that are just living their lives inside of you. And having too many bad bacteria (called gut dysbiosis) can create havoc for your body.

Issues an imbalanced microbiome can contribute to

* Anxiety and depression
* Insulin resistance and type 2 diabetes
* Increased risk of cancer
* Leptin resistance
* Increased hunger
* Slowed metabolism
* Difficulties managing weight
* Irritable bowel syndrome (IBS)
* Inflammatory bowel disease (IBD)
* Small intestinal bacterial overgrowth (SIBO)
* Food intolerances and allergies
* Chronic inflammation
* Autoimmune conditions
* Yeast infections
* Issues in early development

If you develop SIBO – an overgrowth of harmful bacteria residing in the small intestine – symptoms will include bloating, pain, acid reflux, constipation, diarrhea, lethargy, poor concentration and sleep issues.

How to have a balanced and healthy gut microbiome

Things that can be damaging

* Antibiotics
* Hormonal birth control
* Ibuprofen
* High-fructose corn syrup
* Eating a narrow range of foods
* Alcohol
* Smoking
* Lack of sleep

* Stress
* Gluten (if intolerant)
* Dairy foods (if intolerant)
* Consuming foods you are intolerant to
* Steroids
* Irregular bowel movements

Things you can do

* Where possible, limit items on the above list.
* Eat a diverse range of foods.
* Exercise regularly.
* Learn to manage stress.
* Eat probiotic foods or take a probiotic supplement.
* Eat prebiotic foods or take a prebiotic supplement.
* Work with a functional medicine practitioner to run appropriate diagnostic testing, treat pathogens and rebuild any missing keystone beneficial bacterial species.

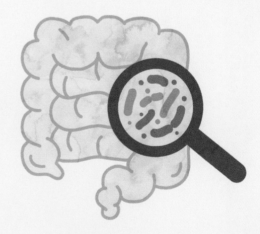

Intention for the week:

MONDAY

SELF-CARE | MEAL PLAN | BODY MOVEMENT

Z^z_z

Today I am grateful for:

TUESDAY

SELF-CARE | MEAL PLAN | BODY MOVEMENT

Z^z_z

Today I am grateful for:

WEDNESDAY

SELF-CARE | MEAL PLAN | BODY MOVEMENT

Z^z_z

Today I am grateful for:

THURSDAY

SELF-CARE | MEAL PLAN | BODY MOVEMENT

Z^z_z

Today I am grateful for:

A single course of antibiotics can disrupt your gut microbiome for a year or more. Consider taking a probiotic and prebiotic to help restore your gut, and eat plenty of probiotic and prebiotic foods.

FRIDAY

SELF-CARE	MEAL PLAN	BODY MOVEMENT
Zzz		

Today I am grateful for:

SATURDAY

SELF-CARE	MEAL PLAN	BODY MOVEMENT
Zzz		

Today I am grateful for:

SUNDAY

SELF-CARE	MEAL PLAN	BODY MOVEMENT
Zzz		

Today I am grateful for:

Fermented foods such as sauerkraut, kombucha and miso contain beneficial probiotic bacteria that increase the health of your gut microbiome and enhance your immune system. Depending on the strain, probiotics can also improve anxiety, depression, heart health, skin conditions, digestive issues and your immune system, and can aid in weight loss and management.

This week, I loved seeing . . .

What on earth is leaky gut?

Leaky gut sounds like it couldn't possibly be a real thing. But it's really just a colloquial name for something that is quite common and often overlooked – intestinal permeability.

The small intestine is where most nutrients are absorbed into your bloodstream via microscopic finger-like tissues that stick out from the intestinal lining. The intestinal lining is formed by cells that sit tightly together, forming a barrier so larger particles of food that haven't broken down, toxins and microorganisms can't enter the bloodstream.

Research is now showing that in some people, the cells in the small intestine are drifting apart, forming gaps in the intestinal lining. This is what is known as 'leaky gut syndrome' or 'intestinal permeability' and just like our microbiome, it can have a massive effect on the health of our mind and body.

Particles that breach the intestinal wall go straight into the gut-associated lymphoid tissue (GALT) where immature immune system cells are forming and growing. The immune system sees these particles as an attack, and to protect you, it releases antibodies. After a while, the immune system can begin attacking its own tissue instead of the particles, triggering autoimmune disease.

What are the symptoms of leaky gut?

Symptoms include fatigue, brain fog, poor memory, headaches, weakened immunity, sugar cravings, digestive issues, acne, rosacea, eczema, weight gain, allergies, joint pain, depression, anxiety and autoimmune conditions.

Why does leaky gut happen?

A component of gluten, called gliadin, causes the release of a newly discovered protein called zonulin. Zonulin can cause the cells in the intestinal wall to open up.

Other things that can cause the cells to open are an overgrowth of candida, too many bad bacteria causing an imbalance in the gut, toxins, inflammation, food allergies, some medications, alcohol, stress and overtraining.

How bad is leaky gut?

Some researchers believe that all autoimmune conditions start with a leaky gut, and therefore, healing your gut is the first line of defence against autoimmune issues. Autoimmune conditions include Hashimoto's, lupus, rheumatoid arthritis and diabetes.

On top of this, leaky gut makes it difficult for the body to absorb nutrients such as vitamin A, magnesium, zinc, vitamin D and calcium. These nutrients are essential to our health. So if you have leaky gut, your body is going to have a difficult time absorbing these nutrients, even if you're taking supplements.

How do you heal leaky gut?

Healing leaky gut is best done with the support of a health practitioner such as a naturopath or functional medicine practitioner. To heal leaky gut, many practitioners embrace the 'four Rs':

Remove: while healing takes place, it is best to remove gluten from your diet along with anything else that can cause irritation or inflammation, such as A1 dairy, alcohol, ibuprofen, processed foods and sugar. Difficult-to-digest foods like steak are also best avoided.

Replace: this is where you introduce gut-healing foods such as bone broth, collagen, fermented foods, coconut products, sprouts, healthy fats, omega-3 fatty acids, and organic fruits and vegetables.

Repair: the addition of repairing supplements such as hydrochloric acid (if stomach acid is low), berberine, zinc and digestive enzymes are essential in restoring the health of your intestinal lining.

Rebalance: finally, you want to balance the microbiome in your gut by taking good-quality probiotic and prebiotic supplements.

WEEK 32

Intention for the week:

MONDAY

SELF-CARE | MEAL PLAN | BODY MOVEMENT

Zᶻᶻ

Today I am grateful for:

TUESDAY

SELF-CARE | MEAL PLAN | BODY MOVEMENT

Zᶻᶻ

Today I am grateful for:

WEDNESDAY

SELF-CARE | MEAL PLAN | BODY MOVEMENT

Zᶻᶻ

Today I am grateful for:

THURSDAY

SELF-CARE | MEAL PLAN | BODY MOVEMENT

Zᶻᶻ

Today I am grateful for:

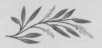

Apple cider vinegar has been shown to improve insulin sensitivity, blood-sugar levels, ovulatory function and gut health; aid in weight-loss; and decrease the LH:FSH ratio.

FRIDAY

SELF-CARE	MEAL PLAN	BODY MOVEMENT

Z^z_z

Today I am grateful for:

SATURDAY

SELF-CARE	MEAL PLAN	BODY MOVEMENT

Z^z_z

Today I am grateful for:

SUNDAY

SELF-CARE	MEAL PLAN	BODY MOVEMENT

Z^z_z

Today I am grateful for:

Prebiotics are a type of fibre that is essential for feeding the good bacteria in our gut. Great food sources are chicory root, Jerusalem artichokes, raw garlic, leeks, asparagus and bananas. Prebiotics can aid in weight loss; reduce our appetite, body fat, insulin levels and inflammation; and improve gut health by helping our good bacteria flourish.

Right now, I feel like my lifestyle is . . .

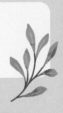

The role of the liver and how you can support it

The liver is arguably one of the most important organs in the body. It performs more than 500 functions in the body and, when stressed, can affect all areas of health. The liver is not a part of the gut but the gut needs the liver to help digest food and the liver needs the gut to remain healthy, or the gut can negatively affect the health of the liver.

* All blood in the body filters through the liver, so it can cleanse the blood of things like toxins and bacteria.
* The liver creates bile, which is needed to break down and digest fats to be used as energy and carry waste away.
* Stable blood-sugar levels are dependent upon the liver.
* The liver creates hormones! And helps us remove excess hormones from the body – this is so important for hormonal imbalance and prevents things like excess estrogen.
* Symptoms of an unhealthy liver include itchy skin, fatigue, bruising, swollen legs and feet, nausea, and loss of appetite. Your GP can help you get blood tests to monitor the health of your liver.
* Non-alcoholic fatty liver disease (NAFLD) affects 1 in 3 Australians and about 25% of people in the USA. It is caused by the liver having a build-up of fat and can lead to serious liver damage.
* Gut dysbiosis and leaky gut can both contribute to liver damage.
* Many of the body's vitamins and minerals are stored in the liver – it's so important we do what we can to protect it.
* Amazingly, the liver can regenerate itself – even when only 25% of healthy liver tissue remains – it's that important. But we need to support it to heal.

WHAT CAN WE DO?

Keep it balanced

Healthy fats are great, but an overload of fat can put too much stress on the liver. So keep those fats balanced!

Limit alcohol

One of the liver's jobs is to break down alcohol. An overload of alcohol can be really stressful on the liver and can cause it damage.

Eat plenty of garlic

Garlic helps to activate liver enzymes that are responsible for removing toxins from the body.

Drink water

Drinking plenty of clean, filtered water whenever you feel thirsty can help the liver do its job.

Include turmeric in your diet

Consuming turmeric in your cooking or taking a supplement with the key compound in turmeric – curcumin – can help to remove carcinogenic compounds from your liver.

Drink dandelion tea

Dandelion tea helps the liver to produce bile.

Talk to your health practitioner about milk thistle supplements

Milk thistle may help to reduce liver inflammation and damage.

Maintain a healthy gut

Ensuring the good bacteria in your gut are supported and healing leaky gut if it is present are essential to the health of the liver.

Intention for the week:

MONDAY

SELF-CARE	MEAL PLAN	BODY MOVEMENT

Z$^{z}_{z}$

Today I am grateful for:

TUESDAY

SELF-CARE	MEAL PLAN	BODY MOVEMENT

Z$^{z}_{z}$

Today I am grateful for:

WEDNESDAY

SELF-CARE	MEAL PLAN	BODY MOVEMENT

Z$^{z}_{z}$

Today I am grateful for:

THURSDAY

SELF-CARE	MEAL PLAN	BODY MOVEMENT

Z$^{z}_{z}$

Today I am grateful for:

Healthy words:
I eat well because my body is important to me.

	SELF-CARE	MEAL PLAN	BODY MOVEMENT
FRIDAY	Zᶻ		
	Today I am grateful for:		
SATURDAY	Zᶻ		
	Today I am grateful for:		
SUNDAY	Zᶻ		
	Today I am grateful for:		

Drink warm or hot water regularly throughout your day to increase blood circulation, release toxins, relieve cramps and aid digestion.

Something I love about my body is . . .

Autoimmune disease

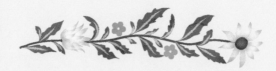

Autoimmune disease might not sound like something you've heard of, but you'll probably find you know someone who is suffering from it.

Autoimmune disease occurs when your immune system begins attacking your own healthy cells. We've included this in the gut health chapter because a major cause of autoimmune disease is believed to be gut health.

There are more than 80 different autoimmune conditions that can be triggered, affecting all different parts of the body and causing all different kinds of symptoms.

Autoimmune conditions affect at least 1 in 5 people worldwide, with rates increasing dramatically in recent years, and research shows that 79% of people suffering from autoimmune conditions are female.

What causes autoimmune disease?

Possible causes include vitamin D deficiency, chronic inflammation, gut dysbiosis, leaky gut and environmental toxins.

Symptoms of autoimmune disease

The conditions that can be caused by autoimmune disease are so vast that innumerable symptoms could be listed. But some common symptoms across many of the conditions include fatigue, joint pain and swelling, skin issues, digestive issues, swollen glands, and recurring fevers.

Treatment for autoimmune disease

Each condition has its own treatment protocol but most conditions will require you to focus on gut health and reducing inflammation.

Some common autoimmune conditions

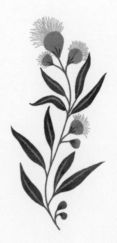

* Chronic fatigue syndrome

* Graves' disease

* Hashimoto's

* Type 1 diabetes

* Psoriasis

* Multiple sclerosis

* Rheumatoid arthritis

* Asthma

* Coeliac disease

* Endometriosis (possibly – yet to be confirmed)

What you can do about it

Whether or not you have an autoimmune condition, we hope that this information really helps you to understand how imperative it is that you prioritise your gut health.

And we hope that this is information you can carry with you for life, so if someone in your circle faces an autoimmune condition, you can help to spread the knowledge that gut health and autoimmunity are linked and can be worked on.

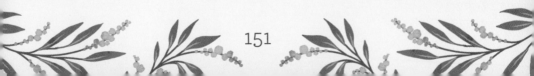

WEEK 34

Intention for the week:

MONDAY

SELF-CARE MEAL PLAN BODY MOVEMENT

Zᶻᶻ

Today I am grateful for:

TUESDAY

SELF-CARE MEAL PLAN BODY MOVEMENT

Zᶻᶻ

Today I am grateful for:

WEDNESDAY

SELF-CARE MEAL PLAN BODY MOVEMENT

Zᶻᶻ

Today I am grateful for:

THURSDAY

SELF-CARE MEAL PLAN BODY MOVEMENT

Zᶻᶻ

Today I am grateful for:

Take a hot bath! Relaxation aside, a hot bath (especially with magnesium salts added) can increase detoxification, reduce inflammation and balance blood-sugar levels, which in turn can improve your egg quality.

FRIDAY

SELF-CARE	MEAL PLAN	BODY MOVEMENT
Zzz		

Today I am grateful for:

SATURDAY

SELF-CARE	MEAL PLAN	BODY MOVEMENT
Zzz		

Today I am grateful for:

SUNDAY

SELF-CARE	MEAL PLAN	BODY MOVEMENT
Zzz		

Today I am grateful for:

Most people know there is a microbiome of bacteria in the gut. But there is also a microbiome in your lungs, your mouth, all over your skin and in your vagina. Yep . . . your vagina is an ecosystem for bacteria. These bacteria help your body to thrive. To support your vaginal microbiome, avoid scented vaginal products, wear natural-fibre underwear, don't douche and consider taking a probiotic.

Something healthy that makes me feel great is . . .

What's your gut telling you?

How are you feeling about the fact that your body is like a spaceship for trillions of bacteria?

☐ Take me home, I'm done

☐ I think it's kinda cool

☐ I'm completely grossed out

☐ I can't really imagine it, so it doesn't affect me

Do you have any symptoms of an imbalanced microbiome? If so, what are they?

_____

_____

_____

Is there anything you're going to do or limit to support the health of your microbiome?

_____

_____

_____

Do you have any symptoms of a leaky gut? If so, what are they?

_____

_____

_____

Will you be talking to your health practitioner about exploring the health of your gut?

☐ Definitely

☐ Maybe

☐ Nah – my gut is tip-top

Will you be taking any steps to support the health of your liver?

_____

_____

_____

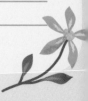

Chapter 7

HELLO
THYROID

he thyroid is a butterfly-shaped gland located at the front of your throat and it is *so* important. If you've heard that it has something to do with metabolism, you've heard right. But the extent to which this beautiful little gland affects your metabolism and every single cell in your body is often glossed over.

The thyroid is the powerhouse of your body. It is showing up for you every single day and absolutely going for it.

Thyroid hormones regulate the body's energy levels and metabolism, body and brain growth, and body temperature.

In this chapter, we're going to paint a picture of just how dedicated the thyroid is to keeping you ticking and what you can do to help protect and improve its health. We will also deep dive on the conditions that can affect the thyroid and how they can be addressed.

Thyroid health is *so* important for living a vibrant and healthy life, and yet there are *so many* people walking around with undiagnosed thyroid conditions. Information about the extent to which the thyroid is involved in our health just isn't being shared and unfortunately, the standard testing issued by many GPs isn't thorough and doesn't align with what is now known about the thyroid. We hope that this chapter will impart knowledge you can use into the future to support the health of you, your loved ones and your community.

How the thyroid affects cellular metabolism

Before we can really dive into how the thyroid affects cellular metabolism, we first need to back up and actually look at what cellular metabolism even is.

WHAT IS CELLULAR METABOLISM? AND WHAT'S A CELL?

Full disclosure – the following information may cause you to sit staring at your hands for upwards of five minutes.

Your entire body is made of cells. As in … it's only made of cells. About 30 trillion cells (oh, and about 130 trillion bacteria … yep, the bacteria living in your body outnumber your own cells).

Cells are the smallest, most basic unit of all living things and they do absolutely everything that is needed for your body to function. They consist of a nucleus, some jelly-like fluid called cytoplasm and a membrane that encapsulates it all.

Some cells live for as long as you do, whereas others live for only a matter of hours – *50 million of your cells die and get replaced every minute!* – oh, and they can replicate themselves.

There are all sorts of cells in the body including skin cells, liver cells, bone cells, egg cells and brain cells, and cells do all sorts of different tasks. Some create stomach acid, some repair wounds, some carry oxygen … the list is long.

For cells to do any of this, they need to take in energy from food and oxygen, and use that energy to perform whatever that cell's job is.

A whole bunch of chemical processes need to happen inside the cell for them to use that energy.

Cellular metabolism is how well the cells perform that process.

If they're guns at it – cellular metabolism is good. If they're struggling, cellular metabolism needs help.

And when cellular metabolism is struggling, it can lead to many, many symptoms and health concerns.

WHAT DOES THE THYROID HAVE TO DO WITH CELLULAR METABOLISM?

Thyroid hormones affect every single cell and function in the body.

The reason for that is, for cells to take in energy and use it to perform their job, they need thyroid hormones. Specifically, triiodothyronine (T3) and thyroxine (T4).

The right amount of T3 and T4 results in a really healthy metabolism – the cells are going to be able to do their jobs without a hassle.

Too much T3 and T4, and the metabolism of the cells is going to go into overdrive. The result? Racing heart, shallow breath, trouble sleeping, weight loss (not always a good thing, people!), anxiety and a whole load of symptoms all across the body that indicate hyperthyroidism/overactive thyroid.

Too little T3 and T4, and the metabolism of the cells is going to become sluggish. Say hello to fatigue, weight gain, dry skin, muscle weakness and a whole bunch of hypothyroidism/underactive thyroid symptoms that so many people are suffering with.

In this chapter, we're going to look at how your body can end up making too little or too much thyroid hormone, and what you can do about it.

For now, what we hope you understand is that cellular metabolism is everything. If your cells can't do their job properly, then something in your body will suffer. A strong cellular metabolism is needed for absolutely every single function in the body, and for your metabolism to be strong, it needs the right amount of thyroid hormone.

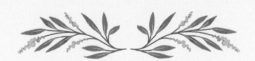

Intention for the week:

MONDAY

SELF-CARE | MEAL PLAN | BODY MOVEMENT

Zzz

Today I am grateful for:

TUESDAY

SELF-CARE | MEAL PLAN | BODY MOVEMENT

Zzz

Today I am grateful for:

WEDNESDAY

SELF-CARE | MEAL PLAN | BODY MOVEMENT

Zzz

Today I am grateful for:

THURSDAY

SELF-CARE | MEAL PLAN | BODY MOVEMENT

Zzz

Today I am grateful for:

FRIDAY

SELF-CARE	MEAL PLAN	BODY MOVEMENT

Z^z_z

Today I am grateful for:

SATURDAY

SELF-CARE	MEAL PLAN	BODY MOVEMENT

Z^z_z

Today I am grateful for:

SUNDAY

SELF-CARE	MEAL PLAN	BODY MOVEMENT

Z^z_z

Today I am grateful for:

The thyroid can develop nodules that are benign or cancerous. Symptoms can include a lump in the neck, difficulty swallowing, hoarseness and neck pain.

This week, I feel proud of myself for . . .

How thyroid hormones work
and how to support them

The thyroid and its hormones work in partnership with two other glands that form the hypothalamus-pituitary-thyroid axis. The HPT axis and the hormones created within it work together a lot like a chain reaction . . .

Hypothalamus

This is a gland in the brain that produces **thyrotropin-releasing hormone (TRH)** when the body's cells require more thyroid hormones. TRH tells your pituitary gland how much stimulation the thyroid gland needs.

Pituitary gland

In response to TRH, **thyroid-stimulating hormone (TSH)** is produced by the pituitary gland, which stimulates the thyroid gland to produce the thyroid hormones T3 and T4.

Thyroid gland

This gland absorbs iodine from food and combines it with an amino acid called tyrosine to produce **T3** and **T4**, in response to the pituitary gland's release of TSH.

T4 is inactive and gets turned into T3 by certain cells in the body.

As we've already covered, T3 and T4 are used by all cells in the body to turn food and oxygen into energy so they can function.

Reverse T3 is a hormone that many health professionals overlook.

Along with converting into T3, a small amount of T4 is also converted into reverse T3. Reverse T3 is an inactive form of T3 but it can be taken up by cells *in place* of T3.

It is believed it exists to act as a barrier to stop too much T3 being taken up by the cells – thus preventing hyperthyroidism/overactive thyroid. It also helps the metabolism to slow down in times of famine.

HOW TO SUPPORT YOUR THYROID HORMONES

* Selenium is needed to convert T4 to T3. Just two or three brazil nuts per day can give your daily dose.
* Iodine is needed to create T4 and T3. Great food sources include roasted seaweed, seafood, dairy foods and eggs.
* Vegetables in the brassica family such as broccoli, cauliflower and kale are known as goitrogens and when consumed raw in large amounts, they can inhibit the thyroid's ability to take in iodine. Lightly cooking brassicas is all you need to do to prevent this happening.
* Consuming carbs and having regular meals is important for thyroid hormones. Low-calorie and fasting diets can trigger the thyroid to go into a state of famine by upping the conversion of T4 to reverse T3, slowing down metabolism. And low/no-carb diets can put stress on the liver, which needs carbs to function and also helps T4 convert to T3.
* Like brassica vegetables, soy foods are goitrogens that can inhibit the thyroid's uptake of iodine. The general consensus seems to be that some soy is fine but a diet based largely on soy may be a problem.
* Colourful fruits and veggies with plenty of antioxidants can help to protect the thyroid from oxidative stress.
* Polyunsaturated fatty acids (PUFAs) such as vegetable oils can inhibit the cellular response to thyroid hormone. Look at preferencing high-quality saturated fats instead – such as coconut oil and ghee.
* High cortisol – produced by chronic stress – can suppress the production of TSH in the pituitary gland, which in turn can lower the production of T4 and T3. It can also increase Reverse T3, reduce the conversion of T4 to T3 and cause cellular resistance to thyroid hormones.

WEEK 36

Intention for the week:

MONDAY

SELF-CARE	MEAL PLAN	BODY MOVEMENT

Z^z_z

Today I am grateful for:

TUESDAY

SELF-CARE	MEAL PLAN	BODY MOVEMENT

Z^z_z

Today I am grateful for:

WEDNESDAY

SELF-CARE	MEAL PLAN	BODY MOVEMENT

Z^z_z

Today I am grateful for:

THURSDAY

SELF-CARE	MEAL PLAN	BODY MOVEMENT

Z^z_z

Today I am grateful for:

'An ounce of prevention is worth a pound of cure.' - BENJAMIN FRANKLIN

FRIDAY

SELF-CARE	MEAL PLAN	BODY MOVEMENT

Z^z_z

Today I am grateful for:

SATURDAY

SELF-CARE	MEAL PLAN	BODY MOVEMENT

Z^z_z

Today I am grateful for:

SUNDAY

SELF-CARE	MEAL PLAN	BODY MOVEMENT

Z^z_z

Today I am grateful for:

Selenium can improve insulin metabolism. It is a powerful anti-inflammatory that can improve mood, depression and anxiety levels; it is essential for a healthy thyroid. Low levels of selenium have been shown to be correlated with increased luteinising hormone and testosterone in the body.

This week, I prioritised my health by . . . .

Underactive thyroid and its various causes

When the thyroid gland does not produce enough T3 and T4, it is known as hypothyroidism or underactive thyroid. Hypothyroidism causes the body's metabolism to slow down, producing many symptoms across the body. Worldwide, it affects about 10% of people assigned female at birth.

SYMPTOMS OF HYPOTHYROIDISM

Symptoms include fatigue, weight gain, depression, anxiety, dry skin, menstrual irregularities, infertility, hair loss, course hair, joint pain, constipation, high cholesterol, memory loss, muscle weakness, sensitivity to the cold, enlarged tongue, puffy face and goiter.

GETTING A DIAGNOSIS

Doctors often look to the symptoms you are experiencing to get an initial idea of the health of your thyroid.

Many doctors will then request a test for TSH only. However, this is not enough information because things like cortisol and inflammation can make TSH appear normal while your thyroid is struggling. It's important to find a doctor who will do the following thyroid tests, to get a full picture of your thyroid health and what exactly is causing the issue: TSH, T4, T3, Reverse T3, anti-TPO, anti-Tg, SHBG and iodine.

CAUSES AND TREATMENTS OF HYPOTHYROIDISM

There are many things that can cause the thyroid to become underactive. Regardless of the cause, a Western medicine doctor may recommend taking a T4 replacement or slow-release T3 or T3/T4 supplement to relieve your symptoms. A natural health practitioner may recommend desiccated thyroid extract to relieve symptoms, which is a natural supplement derived from animal thyroid glands.

The main causes and their treatments are below.

Hashimoto's

Although largely undiagnosed, the main cause of hypothyroidism is Hashimoto's, an autoimmune condition that causes your immune system to attack your thyroid gland, making it less able to produce thyroid hormone.

Hashimoto's can be driven by gut health, stress and certain viruses. A natural health practitioner will consider the following for treatment: a gut-healing diet, stress-reduction, tests for pathogens and infections, prebiotics and probiotics, ashwaghanda, selenium, and D and B vitamins.

Reverse T3

If Reverse T3 levels get too high, the cells won't get enough T3, declining metabolism and leading to hypothyroidism. Reverse T3 can be caused by stress, insulin resistance, inflammation or not eating enough. Determining your cause of Reverse T3 will tell you how to treat it.

Low iodine

Chronically low levels of iodine can cause hypothyroidism. You can increase your iodine levels with a high-quality iodine supplement and by eating seaweed, eggs, dairy and seafood.

Chronic stress

High cortisol can suppress TSH, leading to hypothyroidism. Managing the cause of your stress is key. Check out Chapter 5 for treatments.

Inflammation

Chronic inflammation can damage the cells that produce thyroid hormones. To treat inflammation, check out Chapter 6 about addressing gut health and page 178 about treating inflammation.

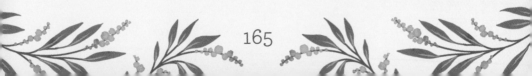

WEEK 37

Intention for the week:

MONDAY

SELF-CARE

Z$^{z}_{z}$

MEAL PLAN

BODY MOVEMENT

Today I am grateful for:

TUESDAY

SELF-CARE

Z$^{z}_{z}$

MEAL PLAN

BODY MOVEMENT

Today I am grateful for:

WEDNESDAY

SELF-CARE

Z$^{z}_{z}$

MEAL PLAN

BODY MOVEMENT

Today I am grateful for:

THURSDAY

SELF-CARE

Z$^{z}_{z}$

MEAL PLAN

BODY MOVEMENT

Today I am grateful for:

Testing for Epstein Barr virus (also known as mono or glandular fever) is important if you are diagnosed with Hashimoto's, because research shows that it causes autoimmune conditions. If Epstein Barr virus is present, a treatment protocol to kill off the virus will be needed.

FRIDAY

SELF-CARE	MEAL PLAN	BODY MOVEMENT

Zᶻ_z

Today I am grateful for:

SATURDAY

SELF-CARE	MEAL PLAN	BODY MOVEMENT

Zᶻ_z

Today I am grateful for:

SUNDAY

SELF-CARE	MEAL PLAN	BODY MOVEMENT

Zᶻ_z

Today I am grateful for:

Iodine is a naturally occurring mineral essential for thyroid health, metabolism, energy production, ovulation and foetal development in the womb. Being deficient in iodine is common, and symptoms include unusual weight gain, muscle weakness, brain fog, fatigue, poor memory, hair loss, dry skin, and heavy or irregular periods. Testing should be done to determine if you are iodine deficient, because iodine should not be supplemented unless necessary.

My favourite moment this week was . . .

Overactive thyroid and how to treat it

An overactive thyroid or hyperthyroidism is diagnosed when your thyroid is found to produce too much T4. This can cause the metabolism to increase to an unhealthy and even dangerous level.

Hyperthyroidism affects about 2% of people assigned female at birth but it is largely undiagnosed.

SYMPTOMS OF HYPERTHYROIDISM

Along with the symptoms below, untreated hyperthyroidism can cause heart disease, osteoporosis and, in rare cases, a potentially fatal complication known as a thyroid storm.

* Insomnia
* Unintentional weight loss
* Hair loss
* Anxiety
* Depression
* Period and cycle issues
* Heat intolerance/hot flushes
* Rapid heart rate, heart palpitations or irregular heartbeats
* Diarrhea

* Hand tremors
* Irritability
* Sweating
* Fatigue
* Increased appetite
* An enlarged thyroid gland (goitre)
* Bulging or uncomfortable eyes
* Muscle weakness
* Fine, brittle hair
* Thinning skin

GETTING A DIAGNOSIS

High levels of T4 and low levels of TSH indicate an overactive thyroid. In saying that, getting the following tests will paint a full picture: TSH, T3, T4, Reverse T3, anti-TPO, anti-Tg, TRAb, TSI, SHBG and iodine.

If blood tests indicate hyperthyroidism, your doctor may request some additional tests such as the radioiodine uptake test, a thyroid scan or a thyroid ultrasound.

CAUSES OF HYPERTHYROIDISM

Hyperthyroidism can be caused by a few rare issues including tumours of the thyroid or pituitary and Plummer's disease. But the most common cause is Graves' disease, which is an autoimmune condition in which antibodies stimulate your thyroid to produce more T4.

HOW TO TREAT IT

People with hyperthyroidism may be offered the solution of removing the thyroid by surgery or by taking radioactive iodine, which shrinks and kills the thyroid gland. Both these options are effective in healing the symptoms of an overactive thyroid. But they do result in the person having the symptoms of an underactive thyroid instead so will need to take synthetic thyroid hormone for the rest of their life.

There are also medications that can be offered to restore thyroid function, with about a 50% chance of remission. However, for some, this medication can damage the liver. Also, one of the medications – methimazole – cannot be taken during pregnancy.

Beta blockers are used to treat any heartbeat symptoms like a racing heart.

Treating Graves' disease

Testing for Epstein Barr virus is important if you have Graves' disease because it can cause autoimmune conditions.

Because Graves' disease is an autoimmune condition, gut health needs to be addressed – see Chapter 6 on gut health for more info.

Unlike with an underactive thyroid, iodine isn't great for Graves' disease so iodine-rich foods like seaweed may need to be avoided.

Other treatments a health practitioner might consider are selenium, L-carnitine, glucomannan and lemon balm.

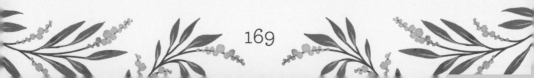

WEEK 38

Intention for the week:

MONDAY
SELF-CARE | MEAL PLAN | BODY MOVEMENT

Zᶻᶻ

Today I am grateful for:

TUESDAY
SELF-CARE | MEAL PLAN | BODY MOVEMENT

Zᶻᶻ

Today I am grateful for:

WEDNESDAY
SELF-CARE | MEAL PLAN | BODY MOVEMENT

Zᶻᶻ

Today I am grateful for:

THURSDAY
SELF-CARE | MEAL PLAN | BODY MOVEMENT

Zᶻᶻ

Today I am grateful for:

L-carnitine is an amino acid supplement that can help with the symptoms of hyperthyroidism (overactive thyroid) and Graves' disease, including nervousness, insomnia, heart rate, fatigue, palpitations and loss of bone mineral density.

FRIDAY

SELF-CARE	MEAL PLAN	BODY MOVEMENT

Z^z_z

Today I am grateful for:

SATURDAY

SELF-CARE	MEAL PLAN	BODY MOVEMENT

Z^z_z

Today I am grateful for:

SUNDAY

SELF-CARE	MEAL PLAN	BODY MOVEMENT

Z^z_z

Today I am grateful for:

Genetically modified organisms/foods (GMOs) including corn, soy, canola, sugar beets have been altered to be resistant to pesticides. GMO consumption has been found to cause hormonal imbalances, sexual dysfunction, lowered immunity, liver and kidney problems, and digestive issues. GMOs may trigger an autoimmune response in the body so many practitioners encourage people with Hashimoto's and Graves' disease to avoid them where possible.

Right now, my relationship with myself feels . . .

Thyroid reflection

Knowing just how important thyroid hormones are for cellular metabolism and the function of your entire body, is there anything you're going to do to support your thyroid health?

_____

_____

These dietary factors can support the thyroid. Circle the things below that you are interested in trying, then talk to a health practitioner to find out if this could be good for your body.

2-3 brazil nuts per day

Eating regularly

Eating plenty of colourful fruits and vegetables

Iodine-rich foods like seaweed and eggs

Eating carbs

Limiting soy

Preferencing saturated cooking oils such as coconut and ghee

Cooking brassicas

After reading about underactive and overactive thyroid, did you find that you had a lot of symptoms of either of the conditions? What were they?

_____

_____

Is your thyroid health something you want to talk to a health practitioner about?

☐ Yes – I need to book an appointment

☐ I'm not sure, I might ask some questions at my next appointment

☐ I know I have thyroid issues and I'm all over it

☐ I know I have thyroid issues but I want to talk to my practitioner about some of the options I've read in this chapter

☐ I think my thyroid is really healthy

Chapter 8

WHEN IT COMES TO NUTRITION
– YOU DO YOU

We are all different. Some people thrive on a plant-based diet. Their acne clears up, they gain mental clarity and their joints stop aching.

Other people reintroduce meat to their diet, and feel nourished and see their cycle become regular, their anxiety decrease and their boobs get bigger.

There is research that supports fasting and research that says it's detrimental. Gluten free? Dairy free? Low carb? Keto? Some see results, others don't.

All this tells us is that there is no single answer to nutrition.

If you are looking for a step-by-step guide to what to eat, we're sorry to say that you won't find that here. It just isn't possible.

What you will find are recipes and info about foods you can add to your diet to support your hormones, and bring more nutrients, nourishment and balance to your body.

You will learn about some key nutritional issues that are affecting more and more people worldwide, and what you can do to avoid or heal them.

And you will learn about how you can find out what *does* work for your body. It's all well and good to hear that a food can be inflammatory – but is it inflammatory in *your* body? Because that's all that matters.

While working through this chapter, we encourage you to keep a record of any food that makes you feel a bit off and any food that makes you feel good.

Super nutrients
and the foods you can get them from

No matter who you are and what dietary approach suits you, one thing is always going to be true – the foods you eat are what ultimately get transferred to your cells and turned into the energy those cells need to do their job. Consuming nutrient-dense foods is the building block of whole-body health, right from the cellular level.

Although we sometimes need supplementation to boost nutrient deficiencies or in place of foods we don't have access to, the easiest way to absorb nutrients is directly from food, so that should always be the goal.

Check out where you can get these super nutrients from and try to incorporate a broad range of these foods in your diet for optimal health.

Zinc – for skin health, hormone balance, fertility and gut health

* Wheat germ
* Oysters
* Meat
* Yoghurt
* Chickpeas

Vitamin C – for collagen, progesterone and immunity

* Citrus
* Strawberries
* White potatoes
* Capsicums/red peppers
* Kiwifruit
* Brussels sprouts
* Turnip greens

Magnesium – for sugar metabolism, inflammation, period pain, thyroid function and mental health

* Nuts
* Seeds
* Raw cacao
* Brown rice

- Dates
- Spinach
- Shrimp/prawns
- Avocado
- Garlic
- Seaweed

Vitamin B12 – for pregnancy, mood, energy, and skin, nails and hair

- Red meat
- Mussels
- Yoghurt
- Eggs
- Nutritional yeast

Vitamin B2 – for thyroid and metabolic function, skin tone and migraine treatment

- Lamb
- Crimini mushrooms
- Sundried tomatoes
- Almonds
- Dairy products
- Eggs

Vitamin B3 – for converting food to energy, inflammation and protecting skin from environmental stressors

- Beef, liver, poultry and fish
- Dairy products
- Eggs
- Avocados
- Whole grains

Vitamin B5 – for breaking down fat, skin hydration and nervous system function

- Beef and chicken
- Organ meats
- Mushrooms
- Avocados
- Nuts and seeds
- Yoghurt
- Oats
- Broccoli

Vitamin B6 – for pregnancy-related nausea, nervous system function, metabolism, hormone balance and acne

- Tuna and salmon
- Beef liver
- Chickpeas
- Poultry
- Papayas
- Oranges
- Bananas

Intention for the week:

MONDAY

SELF-CARE	MEAL PLAN	BODY MOVEMENT

Zᶻ�z

Today I am grateful for:

TUESDAY

SELF-CARE	MEAL PLAN	BODY MOVEMENT

Zᶻz

Today I am grateful for:

WEDNESDAY

SELF-CARE	MEAL PLAN	BODY MOVEMENT

Zᶻz

Today I am grateful for:

THURSDAY

SELF-CARE	MEAL PLAN	BODY MOVEMENT

Zᶻz

Today I am grateful for:

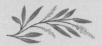

Ginger is antiviral, antibacterial, hormone and blood-sugar balancing and helps to fight inflammation. Try adding a few slices to a cup of hot water with lemon and honey.

FRIDAY

SELF-CARE	MEAL PLAN	BODY MOVEMENT

Zᶻz

Today I am grateful for:

SATURDAY

SELF-CARE	MEAL PLAN	BODY MOVEMENT

Zᶻz

Today I am grateful for:

SUNDAY

SELF-CARE	MEAL PLAN	BODY MOVEMENT

Zᶻz

Today I am grateful for:

There is a Telugu Indian proverb that states, 'Garlic is as good as 10 mothers.' Research has found that garlic can increase the number of calories you burn during daily activities and can decrease the body's production of fat. It can also aid the body in creating the detoxing antioxidant glutathione, and is antiviral and antibacterial. For maximum health benefits, crush or slice garlic, leave it to stand for about 10 minutes, then eat it raw or try to only cook it lightly.

What is something you can do for yourself today to nurture your health?

Chronic inflammation

How it is affected by what you eat and what you can do about it

A cute inflammation happens when you do something like cut your finger and the immune system sends inflammatory cells to the cut to begin the healing process.

Chronic inflammation happens when your immune system is stimulated to send out inflammatory cells on an ongoing basis, which sometimes leads to autoimmune disease.

What causes chronic inflammation?

Stress, untreated injuries and infections, environmental irritants like pollution, and chemicals in beauty and cleaning products can all cause inflammation. A major cause is poor gut health, which is largely driven by the foods we eat.

The reason foods can be inflammatory is because there are certain foods that your body can be sensitive to. And when there's something in your body that your body doesn't really like, your immune system attacks it with inflammatory cells.

It's that simple. But what foods you are sensitive to is individual. For example, gluten can cause an inflammatory response, and yet, some people can consume it and be perfectly healthy.

What are the symptoms of chronic inflammation?

Chronic inflammation can reduce insulin sensitivity (we're going to learn all about insulin in a couple of weeks) and increase cortisol. Those two things alone can cause a cascade of symptoms and conditions including difficulty ovulating, PCOS, autoimmune conditions, hormonal imbalances, thyroid issues, mental health issues, facial hair, acne, hair loss, weight issues, fatigue, joint pain, headaches, and digestive and skin issues.

Your whole body is connected. Healing inflammation can require you to address stressors in your life, your gut health, nutrition, exercise and even things like yeast infections, so it's a great idea to have the support of a health practitioner.

There are definitely a few things you can do to prevent inflammation and heal:

* Embrace anti-inflammatory foods including kale, spinach, almonds, walnuts, blueberries, strawberries, cherries, oranges, broccoli, avocados, turmeric, salmon, mackerel, herring and sardines.
* Heal your gut.
* Talk to a health practitioner about supplements such as turmeric, selenium, magnesium, N-acetylcysteine, dong quai, and peony and liquorice root.
* Work out what foods your body is sensitive to.

HOW TO TEST FOR FOOD SENSITIVITIES

Food sensitivities can irritate the gut, cause leaky gut, create inflammation in the body, cause the immune system to go into overdrive and ultimately lead to autoimmune conditions that can affect every area of the body – from the brain to the thyroid to the ovaries.

There are obvious symptoms of food sensitivities, such as stomach pain and diarrhea, and skin rashes and irritations. But some people can have sensitivities that work in a quieter way, damaging the lining of the gut, causing mental health issues and affecting the thyroid.

There are a few different testing kits you can use to test for food sensitivities, but many of these are not scientifically proven. In saying that, there is science to support some of them, just not enough to convince everyone yet. If you're interested, explore it with a functional medicine practitioner who will recommend the one they think is best.

The simplest way to find your food sensitivities is by doing an elimination diet to see if your body/symptoms respond to the removal of a certain food. Practitioners recommend eliminating the food group for 4–12 weeks.

If a food sensitivity *is* present, people can begin feeling an improvement in as little as a week, although it can also take more than a month to see any results.

At the end of the elimination diet, depending on how you feel, you can begin eating the food again and see how your body responds.

If you try an elimination diet, do so with guidance from a health practitioner.

WEEK 40

Intention for the week:

MONDAY

SELF-CARE | MEAL PLAN | BODY MOVEMENT

Z^z_z

Today I am grateful for:

TUESDAY

SELF-CARE | MEAL PLAN | BODY MOVEMENT

Z^z_z

Today I am grateful for:

WEDNESDAY

SELF-CARE | MEAL PLAN | BODY MOVEMENT

Z^z_z

Today I am grateful for:

THURSDAY

SELF-CARE | MEAL PLAN | BODY MOVEMENT

Z^z_z

Today I am grateful for:

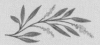

Lemon juice stimulates stomach acid and helps with weight loss, digestion, reducing bloating, absorbing nutrients, boosting collagen and improving inflammation.

FRIDAY

SELF-CARE	MEAL PLAN	BODY MOVEMENT
Z$_z^z$		

Today I am grateful for:

SATURDAY

SELF-CARE	MEAL PLAN	BODY MOVEMENT
Z$_z^z$		

Today I am grateful for:

SUNDAY

SELF-CARE	MEAL PLAN	BODY MOVEMENT
Z$_z^z$		

Today I am grateful for:

In Ayurveda, turmeric is known as the 'friend of women'. Isn't that the best? It can decrease inflammation, improve the complexion, reduce acne, detoxify the reproductive system, help in weight loss and improve insulin resistance.

Three things I love about myself are . . .

Key inflammatory foods - are they affecting you?

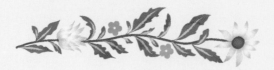

Absolutely any food can be inflammatory for your body – from red meat to sweet potato. Food sensitivities are individual. In saying that, some foods are more commonly inflammatory, and if you have signs of inflammation or conditions like PCOS that can be driven by inflammation, you may want to explore how your body is responding to them.

Common inflammatory foods include sugar, caffeine, alcohol, polyunsaturated fats like vegetable oils, trans fats like deep-fried foods, meat from grain-fed animals, processed meats, nitrates, refined grains, MSG, artificial colours and flavourings, nuts, eggs, and nightshades such as tomatoes and potatoes.

Two of the main foods that can be inflammatory are dairy and gluten . . .

Is dairy for you?

We know consuming dairy is a bit of a controversial topic. From animal welfare to grain feeding, growth hormones and antibiotics – the decision to consume dairy is a complex one. But when it comes to inflammation – the specific component in milk that causes inflammation is a protein called A1 casein, which turns into an opiate in your body. (Are you a 'cheese addict'?)

Some people can pass A1 casein through their body without it reaching their bloodstream, but for people who can't, it can cause an inflammatory response. Signs that A1 casein affects your body include recurring ear infections or tonsillitis as a child, chronic hayfever, sinus infections or dairy cravings.

The good news is some dairy foods are largely free of A1 casein. Jersey cows naturally produce milk without A1 (often sold as 'A2 milk'). Ghee and goat and sheep dairy products are also free of A1 casein.

If you are exploring your sensitivity to dairy, see how your body responds to non-A1 dairy – you may be able to have your cheese and eat it too!

Low-fat dairy products

While we're here talking about dairy . . . For people who have a menstrual cycle, especially if you're trying to conceive, it's best to only consume full-fat dairy.

A huge study has shown that the more low-fat dairy foods there are in a person's diet, the more likely they are to have difficulties conceiving.

Milk is full of hormones. The issue here is that progesterone and estrogen (which are super-important hormones for our cycle) bind to fat. So when fat is removed from dairy, those hormones are removed with it, leaving a low-fat milk filled with unbalanced testosterone. This can prevent follicles from fully maturing in the ovaries, increase testosterone levels and suppress ovulation.

What about gluten?

Ahh gluten, our most beloved staple. Bread, pasta, pizza, baked goods. It's all there. It's all yum.

Humans have consumed wheat for more than 10,000 years – so how is it that so many people become unwell from gluten?

In the 20th century, the processing of wheat was industrialised, and the grains were modified and sprayed with chemicals. What was once a wholefood, which was freshly ground and filled with vitamins, minerals and protein, is now a highly processed filler with little to no nutrients other than carbs.

Symptoms of gluten intolerance include diarrhea and constipation, bloating, abdominal pain, fatigue, nausea and headaches. These symptoms often show up fairly soon after consuming gluten. In saying that, sometimes there is only a low-grade sensitivity that slowly creates an imbalanced microbiome and leaky gut.

Gluten intolerance testing can be done through your GP and begins with a blood test called the Tissue Transglutaminase IgA Antibody Test.

Like all foods you may be sensitive to, you can work with a health practitioner to try eliminating gluten from your diet to see how you feel.

Intention for the week:

MONDAY

SELF-CARE   MEAL PLAN   BODY MOVEMENT

Z^z_z

Today I am grateful for:

TUESDAY

SELF-CARE   MEAL PLAN   BODY MOVEMENT

Z^z_z

Today I am grateful for:

WEDNESDAY

SELF-CARE   MEAL PLAN   BODY MOVEMENT

Z^z_z

Today I am grateful for:

THURSDAY

SELF-CARE   MEAL PLAN   BODY MOVEMENT

Z^z_z

Today I am grateful for:

High in vitamin K, folate, potassium, vitamin C, fibre, antioxidants and healthy fats, avocado is anti-inflammatory and can improve insulin resistance, digestion, weight and heart health.

FRIDAY

SELF-CARE	MEAL PLAN	BODY MOVEMENT

Zᶻᶻ

Today I am grateful for:

SATURDAY

SELF-CARE	MEAL PLAN	BODY MOVEMENT

Zᶻᶻ

Today I am grateful for:

SUNDAY

SELF-CARE	MEAL PLAN	BODY MOVEMENT

Zᶻᶻ

Today I am grateful for:

In Ayurveda, a morning tea made of fresh lime, ginger and honey is said to stoke the digestive fires and detoxify the body, setting you up for a healthy day and optimal gut health. This tea can be tailored to your current condition so it is best to visit an Ayurvedic practitioner to see what is best for you. Also note that in Ayurveda, honey shouldn't be heated above 40°C, so steep the other ingredients then wait until the water has cooled a little before adding the honey.

This week, I loved seeing . . .

Insulin resistance

Insulin resistance is a worldwide epidemic causing health issues that affect an increasing number of people. It is a direct result of our diet and lifestyle.

What is insulin?

Sugars can be found in all foods that contain carbohydrates. These sugars end up in your bloodstream. Insulin is the hormone that prevents your blood-sugar levels from rising too high. It does this by triggering your body to either use the sugars for energy or store the sugars in your cells for later use.

What is insulin resistance?

Insulin resistance occurs when your cells begin to 'ignore' the insulin that has been released. This can happen for several reasons, including poor diet and the use of hormonal birth control. The result is that the cells stop accepting and storing the sugar found in your blood.

When there is excess sugar in your blood, more insulin is released to trigger your cells to store it. However, when there are high levels of insulin in your blood, the cells shut down even more, not wanting to accept toxic levels of insulin and therefore not accepting the sugar. This is a vicious cycle that leads to many symptoms, and can also lead to serious health issues such as Type 2 diabetes.

How can insulin resistance affect us?

Insulin resistance can cause increased testosterone, excess weight around the middle, dark skin patches, skin tags, PCOS, reduced fertility, irregular cycles, acne, facial hair, mood swings, hair loss and leptin resistance (causing you to feel hungry when you're not).

One of the best ways to reduce insulin resistance (and leptin resistance) is by eating a low-glycemic diet, which is based on the concept of the glycemic index (GI). For some people, it is actually all they need to do to completely turn their insulin resistance around.

There are also some great medicinal treatment options that can help with insulin resistance, including myo-inositol and D chiro inositol in a 40:1 ratio, plus magnesium, berberine and chromium.

Aside from eating low-GI foods, the following foods specifically help the body to stabilise blood-sugar and insulin levels.

Resistant starch is a type of carbohydrate that turns into a healthy fat in your large intestine, helps good bacteria grow, and causes a smaller spike in insulin and blood sugar levels than other carbs.

Resistant starch is found in potatoes, sweet potatoes, parsnips, beetroot, oats, pasta and rice. When these carbs are cooked, the starch becomes less resistant, causing higher levels of insulin and blood sugar.

However, once these foods cool down, their levels of resistant starch shoot back up. And when these foods are reheated, the level of resistant starch rises even further.

So, if you are trying to manage your blood-sugar levels, a little hack is to cook these carbs the day before, cool them overnight in the fridge then reheat them the next day.

Fermented foods such as sauerkraut, kombucha and miso stabalise blood-sugar levels by slowing the breakdown of carbohydrates in the gut.

Fibre-rich foods such as flax meal, chia seeds and vegetables help to stabilise blood-sugar levels. Plus they help you feel fuller for longer. People need about 25 grams of fibre every day, so try to add fibre-rich foods to every meal.

Intention for the week:

MONDAY

SELF-CARE   MEAL PLAN   BODY MOVEMENT

Z^z_z

Today I am grateful for:

TUESDAY

SELF-CARE   MEAL PLAN   BODY MOVEMENT

Z^z_z

Today I am grateful for:

WEDNESDAY

SELF-CARE   MEAL PLAN   BODY MOVEMENT

Z^z_z

Today I am grateful for:

THURSDAY

SELF-CARE   MEAL PLAN   BODY MOVEMENT

Z^z_z

Today I am grateful for:

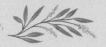

Omega 3 fatty acids can aid in weight loss, reduce testosterone levels, relieve depression, improve egg quality, decrease insulin resistance and reduce menstrual cramps.

FRIDAY

SELF-CARE	MEAL PLAN	BODY MOVEMENT
Z^z_z		

Today I am grateful for:

SATURDAY

SELF-CARE	MEAL PLAN	BODY MOVEMENT
Z^z_z		

Today I am grateful for:

SUNDAY

SELF-CARE	MEAL PLAN	BODY MOVEMENT
Z^z_z		

Today I am grateful for:

Nuts are filled with healthy fats, fibre and antioxidants; can lower the GI of other foods; reduce androgens; and can decrease your risk of diabetes and heart disease.

Right now, I feel like my lifestyle is . . .

Dial up the veg

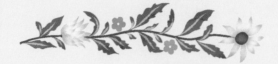

One thing is for sure – vegetables are good. Veggies are packed with fibre and a massive range of vitamins and minerals. Regularly consuming a diverse range of vegetables lowers your risk of cancer and heart disease, improves digestion, and can be a big part of weight management.

The quantity of vegetables we should eat is not really agreed upon, but generally speaking, at least three serves per day is the go-to recommendation. We think having the goal of adding veg to most meals will probably get you over the line and will have the added benefit of turning drab meals into vibrant, balanced, nutritious meals.

Here's a recipe for getting veg into your diet with minimal effort.

EASY-PLEASY GREENS

Low GI, dairy free, gluten free, vegan, anti-inflammatory | Side serve for 4
Cooking time – 20 minutes
These greens easy and are an absolute pleasure.

You can whip them up with next to no thought; they're worthy of the finest of spreads, are entirely customisable and are pure health.

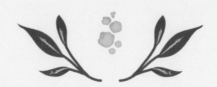

Ingredients

* 2 tbsp fat – ghee, butter, coconut oil, extra virgin olive oil, etc.
* 4 shallots cut into lengths about as long as your pinky finger
* As much garlic as you want
* 1 bunch of broccolini, halved lengthwise (if you've got it in you)
* 1 bunch of asparagus, ends removed
* 1 big handful of green beans (and honestly, just leave the ends on, those ends are a problem for future-you who won't be bothered to care because you'll be in food heaven)
* Salt and pepper to taste
* ½ cup chicken or vegetable stock
* 3 massive handfuls of baby spinach
* Lemon juice to taste

Unnecessary but yum optional extras

* ½ tsp coriander seed powder (if you have it)
* ½ cup toasted flaked almonds
* Goats cheese to taste

Method

1. Heat fat in a large frying pan over medium heat.
2. Spread shallots over the pan then don't touch them. Cook until beginning to brown.
3. Throw in the garlic, broccolini, asparagus and beans (also add the coriander seed powder at this point, if using).
4. Season with salt and pepper.
5. Toss the veggies around then don't touch them until they begin to char.
6. Once charred, add stock and spinach.
7. Cook until veggies are tender (2–6 minutes).
8. Transfer to your most beautiful serving bowl.
9. Squeeze lemon juice all over it.
10. If using, garnish with flaked almonds and goats cheese and enjoy devouring this dish and ignoring whatever it's served next to.

Notes

* You can use absolutely any vegetable you want as long as it can cook in 10ish minutes. Peas, Asian greens, carrots,, capsicums, sprouts, cabbage, Brussels sprouts . . . it's all just great.
* This can all be done on a BBQ and it's arguably better.

Intention for the week:

MONDAY

SELF-CARE	MEAL PLAN	BODY MOVEMENT

Z^z_z

Today I am grateful for:

TUESDAY

SELF-CARE	MEAL PLAN	BODY MOVEMENT

Z^z_z

Today I am grateful for:

WEDNESDAY

SELF-CARE	MEAL PLAN	BODY MOVEMENT

Z^z_z

Today I am grateful for:

THURSDAY

SELF-CARE	MEAL PLAN	BODY MOVEMENT

Z^z_z

Today I am grateful for:

Trying to up your daily veg intake but need to get out the door quickly in the morning? Try introducing whole vegetables requiring zero prep that you can munch on when you're on the go. Whole carrots, snow peas, green beans and cucumbers are all good options.

FRIDAY

SELF-CARE	MEAL PLAN	BODY MOVEMENT
Zzz		

Today I am grateful for:

SATURDAY

SELF-CARE	MEAL PLAN	BODY MOVEMENT
Zzz		

Today I am grateful for:

SUNDAY

SELF-CARE	MEAL PLAN	BODY MOVEMENT
Zzz		

Today I am grateful for:

Organic foods have higher antioxidant levels and lower heavy metal concentrations than regular produce. The antioxidant level is so much higher that eating organic fruits and veggies would be the equivalent to eating 1–2 extra portions of fruit and veg every day. Eating organically can be expensive unfortunately, so focus on making small changes when you can.

Something I love about my body is . . .

Balance it out!

I f we haven't already driven this point home – nutritional requirements are so individual. Something that helps most people's diet, though, is including healthy fats and protein. Carbs are awesome and most experts advise including them at most meals, but it's important to get protein and fat into that meal to balance blood sugar, support healthy hormones and increase nutrients.

Healthy fats are needed for literally every function in the human body – including making hormones. And protein is needed to create amino acids – the building blocks of life needed in everything from digestion to muscle growth.

So here we have a couple of ideas for bringing balance to mealtimes that are often carb heavy . . .

BRINGING THE BALANCE WITH . . . THE GARNISH

Picture some tomato on toast.

Sure, it's yum.

Sure, there are definite nutrients on that plate. But there's also a lot missing from tomato on toast. It's got carbs from the bread, some saturated fats from the butter, and antioxidants and vitamin C from the tomato. But it's not as balanced, nutrient rich or hormone friendly as it could be.

Enter – *the garnish*. Picture this:

Tomato on toast with garnishes

* Ground flax (fibre, omega 3s, protein)
* Sunflower sprouts (vitamins A, D, E and B; folate; potassium; calcium; magnesium; iron)
* Flaked almonds (protein, healthy fats, magnesium, vitamin E)
* Basil (vitamin K, E and C; calcium; manganese, iron)

* Lemon juice (detoxifying, helps absorb iron, vitamin C, immune boosting)

* Goat's cheese, if you eat dairy (selenium, copper, vitamins B2 and B3, calcium)

Can you see how your tomato on toast now looks like a gourmet meal?

And how it has gone from being carb heavy to balanced with healthy fats and protein, and a complex range of vitamins and minerals?

Not only is the meal more nutrient dense, balanced and hormone friendly, it has more flavour and vibrancy. All with foods that require zero prep and can simply be sprinkled on.

The ideas for this are endless and can be applied to so many meals. Everything from soup to ice cream.

Porridge, for example, is nutritious but very carb heavy, which means it will be more likely to create a faster rise in your blood-sugar and insulin levels.

But if you garnish your porridge with nuts, seeds or coconut yoghurt for protein and fat, and fruits and berries for vitamins and minerals, your bowl of porridge becomes balanced, nutrient dense and very hormone friendly.

Other ideas for garnishes include extra virgin olive oil, hemp seed oil, apple cider vinegar, any sprouts, any nuts or seeds, any herbs, and kimchi or sauerkraut.

SNACK-TIME!

Salty, crunchy cravings are a thing and we are here for it.

But have you noticed that a salty, crunchy snack is usually full of carbs? Carbs are awesome but balance is key.

So to spread the love across the macros, we've got a snack that's salty, crunchy, low on the carb-front, and protein and fat heavy.

Introducing . . . spiced pepitas!

In a bowl, combine:
1. 150g pepitas, 1 tsp extra virgin olive oil, ¼ tsp onion powder, ¼ tsp cumin powder and chilli powder, and salt to taste.
2. Toast in a frying pan over medium–low heat, stirring until it just begins to brown. Remove from the heat and snack.

WEEK 44

Intention for the week:

MONDAY

SELF-CARE	MEAL PLAN	BODY MOVEMENT
Zzz		

Today I am grateful for:

TUESDAY

SELF-CARE	MEAL PLAN	BODY MOVEMENT
Zzz		

Today I am grateful for:

WEDNESDAY

SELF-CARE	MEAL PLAN	BODY MOVEMENT
Zzz		

Today I am grateful for:

THURSDAY

SELF-CARE	MEAL PLAN	BODY MOVEMENT
Zzz		

Today I am grateful for:

Healthy fats can balance hormones, improve fertility and help you to maintain a healthy weight. Try making avocados, coconut products, nuts and seeds a part of your regular diet.

FRIDAY

SELF-CARE	MEAL PLAN	BODY MOVEMENT

Z^z_z

Today I am grateful for:

SATURDAY

SELF-CARE	MEAL PLAN	BODY MOVEMENT

Z^z_z

Today I am grateful for:

SUNDAY

SELF-CARE	MEAL PLAN	BODY MOVEMENT

Z^z_z

Today I am grateful for:

Having lots of meals high in carbs without balancing protein and fat may be detrimental – but low-carb diets aren't necessarily the answer. Low-carb diets can increase cortisol levels and inflammation in the body, and increase our risk of insulin resistance and heart disease by five times. It's all about balance!

Something healthy that makes me feel great is . . .

Bring on the breakfast

T
here was a time when breakfast was seen as an essential way to start the day. There was also a time when people put off eating until midday. Both of those times are now.

Yep. Something as simple as breakfast can't even be agreed upon.

There's evidence that kickstarting your digestive system with breakfast is beneficial for your metabolism, blood-sugar levels and a range of other functions.

There's also evidence that fasting until late morning is beneficial for weight loss, blood-sugar levels and, yep, a range of other functions.

There's seriously good research in both camps – so what to do? The answer is always the same – find what works for you. And if you are going to have breakfast, make it a good one.

EGGS POACHED IN TOMATOES

Low GI, gluten free and can be made vegetarian and dairy free
Serves 2 generously | Cooking time – 15 minutes

Ingredients

* 1 tbsp ghee, MCT oil, coconut oil or extra virgin olive oil
* 1 onion, roughly chopped
* 4 cloves of garlic, minced
* 1 cup whatever veggies you have, chopped small (mushrooms, spinach, etc.)
* 1 can of tomatoes
* 1 small can of tuna, chopped ham/ bacon or cannellini beans
* Salt and pepper to taste
* 4 eggs
* 1 handful of basil, roughly torn
* Goat's cheese or nutritional yeast

Method

1. In a lidded frying pan no bigger than 25 cm in diameter, fry onion and garlic until cooked through or browning. Include ham or bacon if using.
2. Throw in veggies and sauté until slightly soft.
3. Add canned tomatoes, tuna or cannellini beans (if using), half the basil, and salt and pepper to taste.
4. Stir all ingredients until combined.
5. Make a well for each egg in the tomato mixture.
6. Crack an egg into each well.
7. Cover and cook until eggs are poached to your preference.
8. Garnish with remaining basil and goat's cheese or nutritional yeast.

CHIA PORRIDGE

Low GI, gluten free, dairy free, vegan | Serves 2 | Cooking time – 15 minutes
Chia porridge is a great meal for hormones and egg health. It's got healthy fats, protein, vitamins and minerals, fibre, and wholefood carbohydrates.

Ingredients

* 400ml can coconut milk
* 4 tbsp chia seeds
* ¼ tsp ground cardamom
* ¼ tsp cinnamon
* ¼ cup flaked almonds
* 1 heaped tbsp sultanas
* 1 tbsp pepitas
* Honey to taste
* Fresh fruit (tropical fruits, kiwifruit, berries, bananas, etc.)

Method

1. Add all ingredients except the honey and fruit to a small saucepan.
2. Bring the mixture to a simmer over low heat.
3. Cook, stirring regularly, until the mixture thickens to a porridge-y consistency. This takes about 10 minutes.
4. Turn off the heat and stir through the honey.
5. Garnish with fresh fruit and serve.

Intention for the week:

MONDAY

SELF-CARE | MEAL PLAN | BODY MOVEMENT

Z^z_z

Today I am grateful for:

TUESDAY

SELF-CARE | MEAL PLAN | BODY MOVEMENT

Z^z_z

Today I am grateful for:

WEDNESDAY

SELF-CARE | MEAL PLAN | BODY MOVEMENT

Z^z_z

Today I am grateful for:

THURSDAY

SELF-CARE | MEAL PLAN | BODY MOVEMENT

Z^z_z

Today I am grateful for:

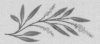

If you're into salad, it can totally be a breakfast food – start with salad vegetables, then add things like eggs, nuts, fruit, cheese and carby veg like roasted pumpkin and parsnips.

FRIDAY

SELF-CARE	MEAL PLAN	BODY MOVEMENT

Z$_Z^z$

Today I am grateful for:

SATURDAY

SELF-CARE	MEAL PLAN	BODY MOVEMENT

Z$_Z^z$

Today I am grateful for:

SUNDAY

SELF-CARE	MEAL PLAN	BODY MOVEMENT

Z$_Z^z$

Today I am grateful for:

High in vitamin D, magnesium, vitamin B3, vitamin B6 and omega 3s, salmon can improve fertility and hormonal balance, and normalise blood-sugar levels.

This week, I feel proud of myself for . . .

Would you like a side of reflection with that?

Just to make sure we're all on the same page – have we made it clear that when it comes to nutrition – we're all different?

☐ Ah yah, you've hit us over the head with it

☐ Sorry, I skimmed over this chapter

Are there any super nutrients you want to focus on getting more of through your diet? What foods will you eat more of to get those nutrients?

_____

_____

Do you have any symptoms of chronic inflammation?

_____

_____

Is there anything you want to do to address or prevent inflammation in your body?

_____

_____

Do you have symptoms of insulin resistance?

_____

_____

Is there anything you want to do to support your insulin levels?

_____

_____

Do you think you eat enough vegetables? If not, what are some ways you could up your intake?

_____

_____

Do you think your plate needs more balance?

_____

_____

After reading this chapter, are there changes you want to make to your overall diet?

_____

_____

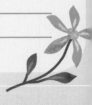

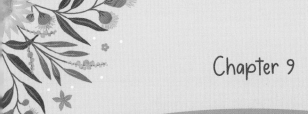

Chapter 9

SELF-CARE PRACTICES THAT ACTUALLY HEAL

'Healing is a matter of time, but it is sometimes also a matter of opportunity.'
HIPPOCRATES

We probably could have just laid that quote down on page 1 and gone home. It's exactly the essence of this journal and it's central to the concept of self-care.

In a world where people are often overworked and free-time is rare, self-care can be a tricky thing to embrace. There's a lot of societal and personal resistance to having 'me time' and downtime.

But self-care isn't selfish. Everyone benefits when your cup is full.

In this chapter, we're going to outline a whole bunch of self-care practices that can improve your health. We hope that, by the end of it, you realise how important it is to give yourself the *opportunity* to prioritise self-care.

The reality is, you're already doing it. Reading this journal and filling it in is a total act of self-care and you should feel super into yourself for being here.

We encourage you to use the monthly habits charts in the back of the journal to add any self-care practices you would like to do daily. If there are practices you'd like to do less regularly than that, we think a great approach is to look at your weekly journal spread and schedule in time across the week for particular practices. It might take you a few weeks to find a schedule that works but it is *so* worth it once you bed it down.

This chapter is luxurious, people – enjoy it!

Self-care rituals for happy hormones

Our hormones are a lens through which we experience life – their rise and fall can make us cycle through feeling happier, more introverted, attractive, energetic, determined, focused, creative . . . the list goes on really.

So it makes a lot of sense to take notice of the signs that our hormones might be a bit out of balance and do what we can to keep them happy.

Signs your hormones might need some love

* Fatigue
* Acne that won't quit
* Difficulty losing weight
* Thin frame with no appetite
* Low libido
* Irregular cycles
* Hair loss

* Notable facial hair
* Difficulty falling pregnant
* Night sweats and hot flashes
* Palpable moodiness
* PMS
* Difficulty sleeping
* Swollen or tender breasts

Self-care rituals that can help

* Get 15–25 minutes of sun every day.
* Eat breakfast within an hour of waking.
* Eat every three to four hours.
* Move your body every day.
* Drink warm or hot water throughout the day.

* Have regular baths in Epsom salts.
* Eat plenty of fibre-rich foods.
* Get seven to nine hours of sleep each night.
* Meditate.
* Drink 2 litres of water every day.
* Practise slow, deep breathing.

Grab a cup!

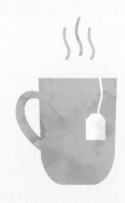

This self-care ritual gets a whole page of its own. It's not just great for happy hormones – this ritual can heal *so many* symptoms and is honestly one of the simplest ways to practise self-care. It's time for a brew.

Medicinal teas you will love

Chamomile
* Antibacterial, anti-inflammatory and liver healing
* Shown to improve sleep and reduce depression

Peppermint
* Antioxidant, antibacterial, antiviral and anticancer properties
* Can relieve nausea, stomach pain and indigestion

Valerian
* Can relax the nervous system
* Can help to induce sleep

Cinnamon
* Anti-inflammatory, anti-spasmodic and blood-sugar balancing
* Can relieve cramps and prevent headaches and stomach issues

Schisandra
* Adaptogenic herb that may help with stress, anxiety and fatigue
* Used in traditional Chinese medicine to relieve symptoms of menopause

Red clover
* Can increase estrogen and progesterone easing menopause symptoms
* Can increase blood flow to the reproductive organs and increase quantity of cervical fluid

Talk to a herbalist about teas that might be right for your body.

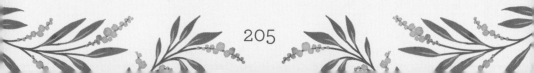

WEEK 46

Intention for the week:

MONDAY

SELF-CARE | MEAL PLAN | BODY MOVEMENT

Z^z_z

Today I am grateful for:

TUESDAY

SELF-CARE | MEAL PLAN | BODY MOVEMENT

Z^z_z

Today I am grateful for:

WEDNESDAY

SELF-CARE | MEAL PLAN | BODY MOVEMENT

Z^z_z

Today I am grateful for:

THURSDAY

SELF-CARE | MEAL PLAN | BODY MOVEMENT

Z^z_z

Today I am grateful for:

Before you can 'set' healthy habits, you have to 'seek' healthy habits. Use this chapter to find habits you love so they can be sustainable.

	SELF-CARE	MEAL PLAN	BODY MOVEMENT
FRIDAY	Zᶻz		

Today I am grateful for:

	SELF-CARE	MEAL PLAN	BODY MOVEMENT
SATURDAY	Zᶻz		

Today I am grateful for:

	SELF-CARE	MEAL PLAN	BODY MOVEMENT
SUNDAY	Zᶻz		

Today I am grateful for:

Self-care is so powerful at healing the mind and body. But it often doesn't happen unless you make time for it. Look at your schedule and find 1- to 10-minute blocks of time – maybe after your shower, before bed or in the car before you get to work – to lock in some time for self-care.

Check in! What could you be doing to focus more on your wellbeing? More 'you' time? More body movement? Connect with friends? Weekend away? Or being immersed in a bath with a book?

The proven benefits of yoga

Originating in India more than 5,000 years ago, yoga is the practice of using meditation, the breath and physical postures to promote health and relaxation. It is more than just stretching – it is a nurturing, detailed health system that has been refined for thousands of years.

Yoga has become a diverse practice presented in a range of styles. Gentle or restorative yoga can relieve stress and reduce cortisol. Yin yoga can increase blood circulation and help joints and muscles function well. Hot yoga can promote the release of toxins through sweat. Avoid hot yoga if you experience a lot of heat, irritability, dehydration, stress or inflammation. Vinyasa yoga can increase fat breakdown and improve insulin sensitivity. Avoid this style of yoga if you have chronic stress or inflammation.

Evidence-backed benefits of yoga

* Reduce cortisol levels
* Lower anxiety levels
* Reduce inflammation
* Fight depression
* Reduce chronic pain
* Improve sleep quality
* Improve flexibility and balance
* Improve lung function in asthmatics
* Relieve migraines
* Improve binge-eating disorder
* Help to lose weight
* Make you stronger
* Reduce delivery time in labour
* Improve libido levels and orgasm
* Decrease all symptoms of PMS
* Improve all symptoms of menopause
* Help with gestational diabetes
* Delay the onset of Alzheimer's
* Help to regulate the menstrual cycle
* Help to balance hormones
* Increase metabolism
* Reduce facial hair
* Improve insulin resistance

Let's get
things pumping

T his is not about getting the blood pumping. This is about an entirely different fluid altogether – lymph. Lymph is a clear fluid made of white blood cells, which pumps around your body in something called the lymphatic system. The lymphatic system is a network of tissues and organs that removes toxins and waste from your cells and carries it out through your urine. It also transports the infection-fighting white blood cells throughout the body.

Another function it has is to move progesterone around your body, so lymph is important for hormone health and fertility. The tricky thing is that it doesn't have its own pump – to move lymph, you need to move your body.

A sluggish lymphatic system can cause toxins and waste to build up in your body, which can lead to a whole bunch of symptoms.

Symptoms of a sluggish lymphatic system

Symptoms include swollen lymph nodes; swollen tonsils; low energy; morning mucous; headaches; brain fog; fluid in the ear; ear popping and ringing; recurrent sore throats; frequent colds and flu; constipation; inability to lose weight; stiffness in the morning; bloating, swelling or heaviness in the arms and legs; pins and needles from sleeping; reduced organ function; spine and shoulder pain; sore breasts; acne; and itchy or dry skin.

Ways to get your lymphatic system moving

Move your lymphatic system with exercise such as swimming, hiking, yoga and rebounding (jumping on a mini-trampoline for just 2 minutes entirely flushes the lymphatic system). You could also try a massage technique called lymphatic drainage massage.

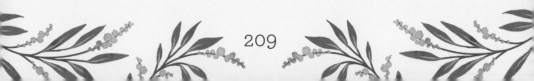

Intention for the week:

MONDAY

SELF-CARE	MEAL PLAN	BODY MOVEMENT

Z Z Z

Today I am grateful for:

TUESDAY

SELF-CARE	MEAL PLAN	BODY MOVEMENT

Z Z Z

Today I am grateful for:

WEDNESDAY

SELF-CARE	MEAL PLAN	BODY MOVEMENT

Z Z Z

Today I am grateful for:

THURSDAY

SELF-CARE	MEAL PLAN	BODY MOVEMENT

Z Z Z

Today I am grateful for:

Use a natural-bristled brush to dry-brush your body. This can improve circulation, reduce cellulite,

FRIDAY

SELF-CARE	MEAL PLAN	BODY MOVEMENT
Z^z_z		

Today I am grateful for:

SATURDAY

SELF-CARE	MEAL PLAN	BODY MOVEMENT
Z^z_z		

Today I am grateful for:

SUNDAY

SELF-CARE	MEAL PLAN	BODY MOVEMENT
Z^z_z		

Today I am grateful for:

There are so many benefits to getting your blood and lymphatic fluid pumping around your body. A super-simple and enjoyable way to do it is to dance. No class needed. Just put on a song or two (or 10) at home and get into it. Try to move every part of your body to really get things moving.

This week, I prioritised my health by . . .

You're never too young (and it's never too late!)
to support your breast health

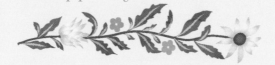

When we hear 'breast health', most of us tend to think of breast cancer. But the health of our breasts can be affected by benign health issues too, such as cysts, fibroadenomas and lipomas. And although it happens more rarely in young people breast issues can affect anyone at any age.

Luckily, like any other part of our body, our breast health can be nurtured and improved. Try incorporating some of the following . . .

* Breast massage – using oil or moisturiser can help and gentle, circular motions are simple and effective in bringing blood circulation to your breasts, helping to prevent and break down any fibrous or cystic tissue.
* Eat about 25 grams of fibre per day, particularly foods high in soluble fibre such as chia seeds, flax seeds, legumes, fruits and vegetables. Fibre has been shown to reduce the risk of breast cancer.
* Get your lymphatic system moving every day through exercise, to help remove toxins from the breasts.
* Get some sun or a liquid vitamin D3 supplement. Vitamin D is arguably the most important vitamin for breast health. Low levels of vitamin D are linked to a greater risk of developing breast cancer, a greater risk of breast cancer recurrence and a lower breast cancer survival rate.
* Using a natural deodorant may support breast health. Some studies have shown that the aluminium found in many standard deodorants may concentrate in breast tissue and cause issues.
* Consider if you really need to take hormonal birth control because this has been shown to increase your risk of breast cancer.

How to do a self-breast-check

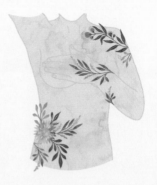

We are all different ... and so are our boobs (if only they told us that in school!). It's important to know what your breasts feel and look like so you notice if something changes.

Research shows that 8 out of 10 lumps found in the breast are not cancerous. However, in Australia, 1 in 7 people with breasts will get breast cancer. Finding it early matters. Luckily, it's very easy to do a self-breast-check!

Three easy steps to check your breasts

It is recommended you do this about once per month.

1. Stand in front of a mirror with your hands by your sides and visually inspect your breasts. Then put your arms in the air and do the same. Once you get used to what your breasts look like, you will be able to notice changes in the contour of your breasts, dimpling of the skin or the shape and colour of the nipple.
2. In the shower, flatten your hand and check the entire breast and armpit area with the flat pads of your three middle fingers. Use different levels of pressure and feel for any lumps, thickening, hardened knots or other changes.
3. While lying down, bend your arm at the elbow and raise it above your head. With your other hand flat like a plate, feel your breast area from your collarbone to your belly and armpit. Feel for lumps like you did in the shower but also squeeze the nipple to check for discharge or lumps.

If you find something, don't panic – 8 out of 10 times, it isn't cancer. Call your doctor and book an appointment. Your doctor will check your breasts themselves. If they too find something, they will recommend you get either a mammogram, ultrasound, MRI or biopsy.

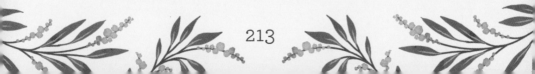

WEEK 48

Intention for the week:

MONDAY

SELF-CARE | MEAL PLAN | BODY MOVEMENT

Zᶻz

Today I am grateful for:

TUESDAY

SELF-CARE | MEAL PLAN | BODY MOVEMENT

Zᶻz

Today I am grateful for:

WEDNESDAY

SELF-CARE | MEAL PLAN | BODY MOVEMENT

Zᶻz

Today I am grateful for:

THURSDAY

SELF-CARE | MEAL PLAN | BODY MOVEMENT

Zᶻz

Today I am grateful for:

About 50% of the global population are deficient in vitamin D. Vitamin D is essential for fertility; weight management; mental health; skin, bone and heart health; and metabolism. Vitamin D deficiency is correlated with less IVF success. Maintain your vitamin D levels with 15 minutes of sunshine each day.

FRIDAY

SELF-CARE	MEAL PLAN	BODY MOVEMENT

Zᶻz

Today I am grateful for:

SATURDAY

SELF-CARE	MEAL PLAN	BODY MOVEMENT

Zᶻz

Today I am grateful for:

SUNDAY

SELF-CARE	MEAL PLAN	BODY MOVEMENT

Zᶻz

Today I am grateful for:

In Ayurveda, it is encouraged to do a daily full-body self-massage with oil. Studies have shown it to decrease stress, improve sleep quality and enhance your overall quality of life. It can also support the nervous system, improve lymph and blood circulation, tone muscles, keep skin soft and hair strong, increase longevity, and slow the signs of aging. See an Ayurvedic practitioner to get a medicinal herbal oil tailored to you.

My favourite moment this week was . . .

Where's the vitality at?

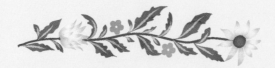

Yet another 'taboo' topic is on the agenda . . . Libido. AKA, sex drive. When it comes to sex, some people are up for it anytime, anywhere. Others can take it or leave it. For some, it's like 10-pin bowling – entirely unappealing until you're actually there and you remember that it's great. And for others, sex and feeling sexy are far from their radar.

The interesting thing is, because talking about sex and libido is so taboo, many people are walking around with a low libido, wishing it was healthier but completely unaware that there might be a reason why.

If your sex drive is stalling and you wish it wasn't, check out these possible causes and have a chat to a health professional about it.

Wanting a sex drive isn't something to be ashamed of and it doesn't mean you need to find anyone else to enjoy it with. A healthy libido is a sign of good health and a low libido is often a message from your body that something might be up. So listen to your body and talk to your health professional.

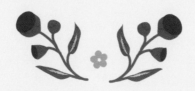

Reasons for a low libido

- Pain during sex
- Antidepressants
- The pill
- Alcohol and cigarettes
- Medical conditions such as cancer, diabetes and arthritis
- Fatigue
- Menopause
- Low estrogen
- Pregnancy and breastfeeding
- Anxiety or depression
- Low self-esteem
- Previous abuse
- Previous negative sexual experiences
- Lack of connection or trust with your sexual partner
- PMS
- Endometriosis
- Pelvic inflammatory disease
- Prolapse
- Haemorrhoids
- Anaemia
- Kidney failure
- Infections (such as thrush or urinary tract)
- Hypothyroidism
- Chronic pain
- Low testosterone
- Stress

WEEK 49

Intention for the week:

MONDAY

SELF-CARE | MEAL PLAN | BODY MOVEMENT

Z^z_z

Today I am grateful for:

TUESDAY

SELF-CARE | MEAL PLAN | BODY MOVEMENT

Z^z_z

Today I am grateful for:

WEDNESDAY

SELF-CARE | MEAL PLAN | BODY MOVEMENT

Z^z_z

Today I am grateful for:

THURSDAY

SELF-CARE | MEAL PLAN | BODY MOVEMENT

Z^z_z

Today I am grateful for:

Try oil pulling. Swish coconut or sesame oil around in your mouth for 5–15 minutes. After just a few days, you may notice your teeth are whiter, and feel smoother and cleaner. It is also said to remove toxins and bacteria from your mouth.

FRIDAY

SELF-CARE	MEAL PLAN	BODY MOVEMENT

Z^zz

Today I am grateful for:

SATURDAY

SELF-CARE	MEAL PLAN	BODY MOVEMENT

Z^zz

Today I am grateful for:

SUNDAY

SELF-CARE	MEAL PLAN	BODY MOVEMENT

Z^zz

Today I am grateful for:

Give your skin some attention and love with a homemade facial scrub. A simple combo of milk and brown sugar smells great, feels great and is incredibly healing for sun-damaged skin.

Right now, my relationship with myself feels . . .

Beauty products
The 'dirty dozen' of ingredients

Believe it or not, many beauty products are laden with chemicals that can do everything from increase your risk of breast cancer to mess with your hormones and damage your liver.

Below is a list of the 'dirty dozen' that you want to avoid if you can. Take a photo of this list and crosscheck it the next time you're out buying beauty products.

BHA (butylated hydroxyanisole) and BHT (butylated hydroxytoluene)

* Synthetic antioxidants
* Carcinogenic
* May cause liver damage

Coal tar dyes

* Look for p-Phenylenediamine or 'C.I' followed by five numbers
* Anti-dandruff and colorant
* Can be filled with toxic heavy metals
* Carcinogenic
* Possibly cancer causing

Ethanolamines (MEA/DEA/TEA)

* pH adjuster
* Hormone disrupting
* Can inhibit foetal brain development

Phthalates (DBP, DEHP, DEP, etc.)

* Helps fragrance stick to skin
* Hormone disrupting
* May cause birth defects

Formaldehyde-releasing preservatives

* Look for quaternium-15, DMDM hydantoin, methenamine, imidazolidinyl urea, diazolidinyl urea, sodium hydroxymethylglycinate, 2-bromo-2-nitropropane-1 and 3 diol (Bronopol)
* Carcinogenic
* Linked to asthma

Parabens

* Look for propylparaben, methylparaben and butylparaben
* Common preservative
* Linked to breast cancer
* Hormone disrupting

Synthetic fragrance/perfumes

* Linked to cancer
* Hormone disrupting
* May trigger allergies and asthma

PEG compounds

* Thickener and softener
* Carcinogenic
* Laxative

Mineral oil, paraffin, and petrolatum

* May cause cancer
* Skin irritations and allergies
* Carcinogenic
* Slow cellular development

Oxybenzone

* Sunscreen agent
* Cellular damage
* Hormone disrupting
* Irritation and allergies

Sodium laureth sulfate (SLS) and sodium laureth ether sulfate (SLES)

* Cleanser and emulsifier
* Carcinogenic
* Irritation and allergies

Triclosan

* Preservative
* Hormone disrupting
* May contribute to antibiotic-resistant bacteria
* Antimicrobial pesticide

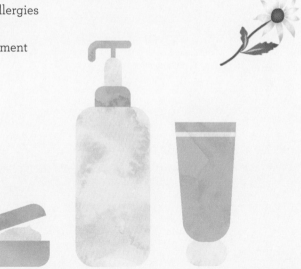

Intention for the week:

MONDAY

SELF-CARE

MEAL PLAN

BODY MOVEMENT

Z^z_z

Today I am grateful for:

TUESDAY

SELF-CARE

MEAL PLAN

BODY MOVEMENT

Z^z_z

Today I am grateful for:

WEDNESDAY

SELF-CARE

MEAL PLAN

BODY MOVEMENT

Z^z_z

Today I am grateful for:

THURSDAY

SELF-CARE

MEAL PLAN

BODY MOVEMENT

Z^z_z

Today I am grateful for:

Healthy words:
Each day, I become a better version of myself.

FRIDAY

SELF-CARE	MEAL PLAN	BODY MOVEMENT

Z^z_z

Today I am grateful for:

SATURDAY

SELF-CARE	MEAL PLAN	BODY MOVEMENT

Z^z_z

Today I am grateful for:

SUNDAY

SELF-CARE	MEAL PLAN	BODY MOVEMENT

Z^z_z

Today I am grateful for:

Use your favourite oil or moisturiser to give yourself a hand massage. So underrated – but so good! Plus, according to many modalities, our hands are filled with pressure points that correspond with our whole body, so hand massage is practically medicinal.

What is something you can do for yourself today to nurture your health?

The importance of sleep

Sleep is one of the most powerful elements of human life. Yet many of us struggle to prioritise it. And when we are having sleep issues like night waking or trouble falling asleep, it can feel really hard to address the issue.

WHY YOU NEED A GOOD NIGHT'S SLEEP

Poor sleep can lead to increased cortisol levels, diabetes, PCOS, Cushing's syndrome, weight gain, low libido, anxiety, depression, irregular cycles, insulin resistance, increased testosterone, sugar cravings and difficulties detoxifying.

WAYS TO IMPROVE YOUR SLEEP QUALITY

* Go to bed by 10 pm (11 pm latest)
* Get 7–9 hours of sleep
* Sleep and wake at the same time every day
* Use blue-light glasses or a blue-light filter
* Don't do cardio within three hours of bedtime
* Reduce caffeine, nicotine and alcohol consumption
* Have a hot bath right before bed
* Keep the bedroom free from devices
* Get 2–10 minutes of morning sun and dim the lights at night

Don't knock it 'til you've coloured it

To some people, colouring-in might seem childish or pointless. But amazingly, research has found that colouring-in can cause drastic and immediate reductions in stress and anxiety. These things are all about the individual , though, and you can't know if something is helpful until you give it a try. So if you're feeling that anxious tension, have a colour and see how you feel…

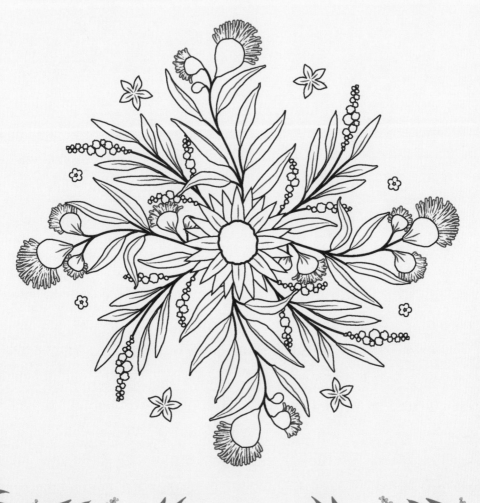

Intention for the week:

MONDAY

SELF-CARE	MEAL PLAN	BODY MOVEMENT

Z^z_z

Today I am grateful for:

TUESDAY

SELF-CARE	MEAL PLAN	BODY MOVEMENT

Z^z_z

Today I am grateful for:

WEDNESDAY

SELF-CARE	MEAL PLAN	BODY MOVEMENT

Z^z_z

Today I am grateful for:

THURSDAY

SELF-CARE	MEAL PLAN	BODY MOVEMENT

Z^z_z

Today I am grateful for:

Take off your shoes and go for a barefoot walk on this beautiful planet of ours – it's called 'earthing'. Research is showing that, by passing free electrons from the earth into your body through your skin, earthing can reduce free radicals and inflammation and improve sleep.

FRIDAY

SELF-CARE	MEAL PLAN	BODY MOVEMENT
Z^z_z		

Today I am grateful for:

SATURDAY

SELF-CARE	MEAL PLAN	BODY MOVEMENT
Z^z_z		

Today I am grateful for:

SUNDAY

SELF-CARE	MEAL PLAN	BODY MOVEMENT
Z^z_z		

Today I am grateful for:

Do you have five minutes free? Maybe just after your shower or before you start work? Even if you only have two minutes, you can maximise that time by doing some meditation. There are some amazing, free apps out there with different meditation styles of different lengths.

Who is someone you love who you haven't spoken to in ages? Get in touch with them this week . . .

Yoga poses that just feel damn good

Crocodile pose

Lengthens the spine, decreasing pressure in the lower back. Feels amazing, especially if you sit a lot.

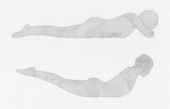

Rag doll pose

Lengthens the spine, hamstrings, and neck. Gives a big sense of 'letting go'.

Wide-legged seated forward fold

This pose stretches so many parts of the legs and groin, and naturally slows you down. Feels good physically and creates a sense of calm.

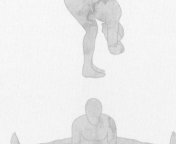

Knees-to-chest pose

With a little rocking, this is becomes a back massage. It also massages your abdominal organs, eases tension in the lower back and can reduce bloating.

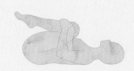

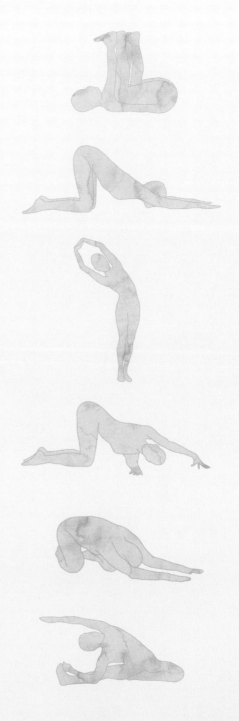

Happy baby pose

Releasing tension in the hips, this absolute winner of a pose also delivers on the back massage.

Extended puppy pose

Opens the chest, stretches the spine and shoulders, and feels sensational.

Side mountain pose

Improves posture and balance and gives a fantastic stretch to the side of the upper body.

Thread the needle pose

Relieves serious tension in the upper body and shoulders.

Child's pose with side stretch

Stretches the muscles around the ribs and relieves tension in the mid and upper back.

Revolved head-to-knee pose

Good for headaches, insomnia, fatigue and digestion, this pose has almost as many benefits as it does units of 'oh yeah'.

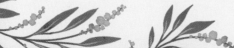

Intention for the week:

MONDAY

SELF-CARE	MEAL PLAN	BODY MOVEMENT

Z^z_z

Today I am grateful for:

TUESDAY

SELF-CARE	MEAL PLAN	BODY MOVEMENT

Z^z_z

Today I am grateful for:

WEDNESDAY

SELF-CARE	MEAL PLAN	BODY MOVEMENT

Z^z_z

Today I am grateful for:

THURSDAY

SELF-CARE	MEAL PLAN	BODY MOVEMENT

Z^z_z

Today I am grateful for:

'Happiness is the highest form of health.'
– DALAI LAMA

FRIDAY

SELF-CARE	MEAL PLAN	BODY MOVEMENT

Zᶻᶻ

Today I am grateful for:

SATURDAY

SELF-CARE	MEAL PLAN	BODY MOVEMENT

Zᶻᶻ

Today I am grateful for:

SUNDAY

SELF-CARE	MEAL PLAN	BODY MOVEMENT

Zᶻᶻ

Today I am grateful for:

Deep breathing exercises promote deep relaxation and hormonal balance, and help to put you into a state of rest and digest. Let's end these 52 weeks of self-care with just a few slow, deep breaths as many times as possible throughout the day. And when you do it, try to take the moment to reflect on how your health has progressed over the past 12 months.

How do I feel having prioritised my health for a whole year?

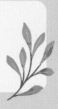

Feeling relaxed yet?

Knowing there are some powerful self-care practices that take just a few minutes to do, are there any times of day that you could slip some self-care into?

_____

_____

Are there any self-care practices you're going to embrace that are good for keeping hormones happy?

_____

_____

Medicinal teas are an easy, healing way to practice self-care – are there any teas you're going to try out?

_____

_____

Do you have symptoms of a sluggish lymphatic system? If so – will you be adding any practices in to get it pumping?

| Exercise | Dancing | Lymphatic drainage massage |

| Rebounding | Body Brushing |

Are you going to begin doing breast checks?

☐ 100%
☐ I already do it

Were you surprised to see how damaging some beauty product ingredients are?

☐ So surprised! I'm going to switch over to healthier brands
☐ I was surprised but I'm fine with it
☐ Not at all, I use really clean products already

How's your sleep? Do you need more or less? Are there any practices you will bring to your sleep routine to improve it?

_____

_____

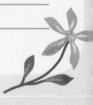

YOUR MONTHLY CHARTS

This section contains 12 months of charts you can fill in to help you track and understand your body. You'll find further explanations below.

Symptoms and treatments chart

Use each section of this chart to track a symptom, such as stress, moodiness, acne or back pain. Each day, mark how the symptom is presenting – at its worst, bad, average, good or at its best. In the section at the bottom of the chart, write any treatment method you are using and the date you start it.

Cycle chart

Understanding your cycle and when/if you are ovulating is a great way to begin understanding your body. Use this chart to track your basal body temperature, period, cervical fluid, and cervical position and texture. And if you are trying to conceive, track when you are having sex.

Daily habits chart

Make a list of the things you want to achieve every day and tick them off each night. This is the perfect place to list supplements and self-care practices.

Weight chart

You can use this simple and customisable chart to track your weight. If tracking your weight doesn't make you feel good – just skip this one.

At the end of this section you will also find a chart for recording test results and a chart for recording how you experience each phase of your cycle.

Symptoms & treatments

Month:

SYMPTOM:

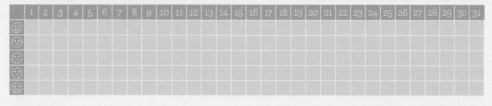

	1	2	3	4	5	6	7	8	9	10	11	12	13	14	15	16	17	18	19	20	21	22	23	24	25	26	27	28	29	30	31

SYMPTOM:

	1	2	3	4	5	6	7	8	9	10	11	12	13	14	15	16	17	18	19	20	21	22	23	24	25	26	27	28	29	30	31

SYMPTOM:

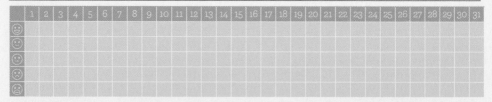

	1	2	3	4	5	6	7	8	9	10	11	12	13	14	15	16	17	18	19	20	21	22	23	24	25	26	27	28	29	30	31

SYMPTOM:

	1	2	3	4	5	6	7	8	9	10	11	12	13	14	15	16	17	18	19	20	21	22	23	24	25	26	27	28	29	30	31

SYMPTOM:

	1	2	3	4	5	6	7	8	9	10	11	12	13	14	15	16	17	18	19	20	21	22	23	24	25	26	27	28	29	30	31

SYMPTOM:

	1	2	3	4	5	6	7	8	9	10	11	12	13	14	15	16	17	18	19	20	21	22	23	24	25	26	27	28	29	30	31
😀																															
🙂																															
😐																															
🙁																															
😣																															

SYMPTOM:

	1	2	3	4	5	6	7	8	9	10	11	12	13	14	15	16	17	18	19	20	21	22	23	24	25	26	27	28	29	30	31
😀																															
🙂																															
😐																															
🙁																															
😣																															

SYMPTOM:

	1	2	3	4	5	6	7	8	9	10	11	12	13	14	15	16	17	18	19	20	21	22	23	24	25	26	27	28	29	30	31
😀																															
🙂																															
😐																															
🙁																															
😣																															

SYMPTOM:

	1	2	3	4	5	6	7	8	9	10	11	12	13	14	15	16	17	18	19	20	21	22	23	24	25	26	27	28	29	30	31
😀																															
🙂																															
😐																															
🙁																															
😣																															

TREATMENT STARTED: **A**

B   C

D   E

F   G

	1	2	3	4	5	6	7	8	9	10	11	12	13	14	15	16	17	18	19	20	21	22	23	24	25	26	27	28	29	30	31
A																															
B																															
C																															
D																															
E																															
F																															
G																															

Habits

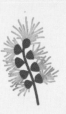

Month:

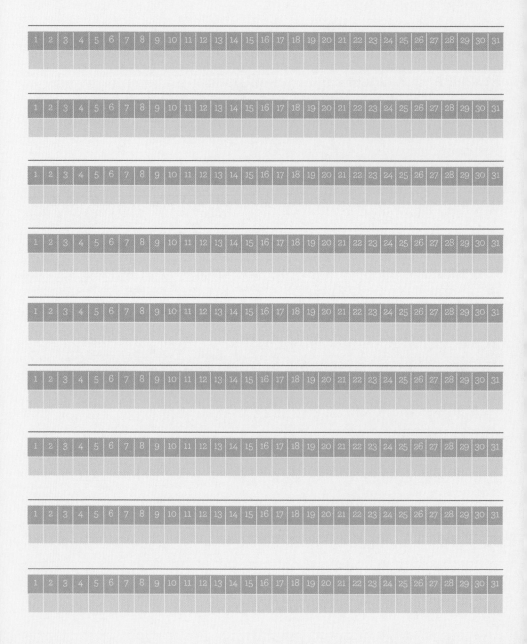

| 1 | 2 | 3 | 4 | 5 | 6 | 7 | 8 | 9 | 10 | 11 | 12 | 13 | 14 | 15 | 16 | 17 | 18 | 19 | 20 | 21 | 22 | 23 | 24 | 25 | 26 | 27 | 28 | 29 | 30 | 31 |

| 1 | 2 | 3 | 4 | 5 | 6 | 7 | 8 | 9 | 10 | 11 | 12 | 13 | 14 | 15 | 16 | 17 | 18 | 19 | 20 | 21 | 22 | 23 | 24 | 25 | 26 | 27 | 28 | 29 | 30 | 31 |

| 1 | 2 | 3 | 4 | 5 | 6 | 7 | 8 | 9 | 10 | 11 | 12 | 13 | 14 | 15 | 16 | 17 | 18 | 19 | 20 | 21 | 22 | 23 | 24 | 25 | 26 | 27 | 28 | 29 | 30 | 31 |

| 1 | 2 | 3 | 4 | 5 | 6 | 7 | 8 | 9 | 10 | 11 | 12 | 13 | 14 | 15 | 16 | 17 | 18 | 19 | 20 | 21 | 22 | 23 | 24 | 25 | 26 | 27 | 28 | 29 | 30 | 31 |

| 1 | 2 | 3 | 4 | 5 | 6 | 7 | 8 | 9 | 10 | 11 | 12 | 13 | 14 | 15 | 16 | 17 | 18 | 19 | 20 | 21 | 22 | 23 | 24 | 25 | 26 | 27 | 28 | 29 | 30 | 31 |

| 1 | 2 | 3 | 4 | 5 | 6 | 7 | 8 | 9 | 10 | 11 | 12 | 13 | 14 | 15 | 16 | 17 | 18 | 19 | 20 | 21 | 22 | 23 | 24 | 25 | 26 | 27 | 28 | 29 | 30 | 31 |

| 1 | 2 | 3 | 4 | 5 | 6 | 7 | 8 | 9 | 10 | 11 | 12 | 13 | 14 | 15 | 16 | 17 | 18 | 19 | 20 | 21 | 22 | 23 | 24 | 25 | 26 | 27 | 28 | 29 | 30 | 31 |

| 1 | 2 | 3 | 4 | 5 | 6 | 7 | 8 | 9 | 10 | 11 | 12 | 13 | 14 | 15 | 16 | 17 | 18 | 19 | 20 | 21 | 22 | 23 | 24 | 25 | 26 | 27 | 28 | 29 | 30 | 31 |

| 1 | 2 | 3 | 4 | 5 | 6 | 7 | 8 | 9 | 10 | 11 | 12 | 13 | 14 | 15 | 16 | 17 | 18 | 19 | 20 | 21 | 22 | 23 | 24 | 25 | 26 | 27 | 28 | 29 | 30 | 31 |

Weight

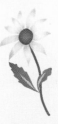

Month:

	1	2	3	4	5	6	7	8	9	10	11	12	13	14	15	16	17	18	19	20	21	22	23	24	25	26	27	28	29	30	31
W																															
E																															
I																															
G																															
H																															
T																															

Cycle tracking

Month: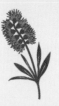

TEMPERATURE	1	2	3	4	5	6	7	8	9	10	11	12	13	14
37.30°C/99.4°F														
37.25°C/99.3°F														
37.20°C/99.2°F														
37.15°C/99.1°F														
37.10°C/99.0°F														
37.05°C/98.9°F														
37.00°C/98.8°F														
36.95°C/98.7°F														
36.90°C/98.6°F														
36.85°C/98.5°F														
36.80°C/98.4°F														
36.75°C/98.3°F														
36.70°C/98.2°F														
36.65°C/98.1°F														
36.60°C/98.0°F														
36.55°C/97.9°F														
36.50°C/97.8°F														
36.45°C/97.7°F														
36.40°C/97.6°F														
36.35°C/97.5°F														
36.30°C/97.4°F														
36.25°C/97.3°F														
36.20°C/97.2°F														
36.15°C/97.1°F														
36.10°C/97.0°F														
36.05°C/96.9°F														
36.00°C/96.8°F														
35.95°C/96.7°F														
35.90°C/96.6°F														

Cervical fluid														
Cervical position														
Cervical texture														
Sex														
Ovulation test														
Pregnancy test														
Period														
Day of cycle														

CERVICAL FLUID: **S** – Sticky   **C** – Creamy   **W** – Watery   **E** – Egg white

CERVICAL POSITION: **L** – Low   **M** – Medium   **H** – High

CERVICAL TEXTURE: **S** – Soft   **M** – Medium   **F** – Firm

15	16	17	18	19	20	21	22	23	24	25	26	27	28	29	30	31

Symptoms & treatments

Month:

SYMPTOM:

	1	2	3	4	5	6	7	8	9	10	11	12	13	14	15	16	17	18	19	20	21	22	23	24	25	26	27	28	29	30	31
😀																															
🙂																															
😐																															
🙁																															
😣																															

SYMPTOM:

	1	2	3	4	5	6	7	8	9	10	11	12	13	14	15	16	17	18	19	20	21	22	23	24	25	26	27	28	29	30	31
😀																															
🙂																															
😐																															
🙁																															
😣																															

SYMPTOM:

	1	2	3	4	5	6	7	8	9	10	11	12	13	14	15	16	17	18	19	20	21	22	23	24	25	26	27	28	29	30	31
😀																															
🙂																															
😐																															
🙁																															
😣																															

SYMPTOM:

	1	2	3	4	5	6	7	8	9	10	11	12	13	14	15	16	17	18	19	20	21	22	23	24	25	26	27	28	29	30	31
😀																															
🙂																															
😐																															
🙁																															
😣																															

SYMPTOM:

	1	2	3	4	5	6	7	8	9	10	11	12	13	14	15	16	17	18	19	20	21	22	23	24	25	26	27	28	29	30	31
😀																															
🙂																															
😐																															
🙁																															
😣																															

SYMPTOM: _____

	1	2	3	4	5	6	7	8	9	10	11	12	13	14	15	16	17	18	19	20	21	22	23	24	25	26	27	28	29	30	31
☺																															
☺																															
☺																															
☹																															
☹																															

SYMPTOM: _____

	1	2	3	4	5	6	7	8	9	10	11	12	13	14	15	16	17	18	19	20	21	22	23	24	25	26	27	28	29	30	31
☺																															
☺																															
☺																															
☹																															
☹																															

SYMPTOM: _____

	1	2	3	4	5	6	7	8	9	10	11	12	13	14	15	16	17	18	19	20	21	22	23	24	25	26	27	28	29	30	31
☺																															
☺																															
☺																															
☹																															
☹																															

SYMPTOM: _____

	1	2	3	4	5	6	7	8	9	10	11	12	13	14	15	16	17	18	19	20	21	22	23	24	25	26	27	28	29	30	31
☺																															
☺																															
☺																															
☹																															
☹																															

TREATMENT STARTED: **A** _____

B _____ C _____

D _____ E _____

F _____ G _____

	1	2	3	4	5	6	7	8	9	10	11	12	13	14	15	16	17	18	19	20	21	22	23	24	25	26	27	28	29	30	31
A																															
B																															
C																															
D																															
E																															
F																															
G																															

Habits

Month:

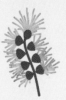

1	2	3	4	5	6	7	8	9	10	11	12	13	14	15	16	17	18	19	20	21	22	23	24	25	26	27	28	29	30	31

1	2	3	4	5	6	7	8	9	10	11	12	13	14	15	16	17	18	19	20	21	22	23	24	25	26	27	28	29	30	31

1	2	3	4	5	6	7	8	9	10	11	12	13	14	15	16	17	18	19	20	21	22	23	24	25	26	27	28	29	30	31

1	2	3	4	5	6	7	8	9	10	11	12	13	14	15	16	17	18	19	20	21	22	23	24	25	26	27	28	29	30	31

1	2	3	4	5	6	7	8	9	10	11	12	13	14	15	16	17	18	19	20	21	22	23	24	25	26	27	28	29	30	31

1	2	3	4	5	6	7	8	9	10	11	12	13	14	15	16	17	18	19	20	21	22	23	24	25	26	27	28	29	30	31

1	2	3	4	5	6	7	8	9	10	11	12	13	14	15	16	17	18	19	20	21	22	23	24	25	26	27	28	29	30	31

1	2	3	4	5	6	7	8	9	10	11	12	13	14	15	16	17	18	19	20	21	22	23	24	25	26	27	28	29	30	31

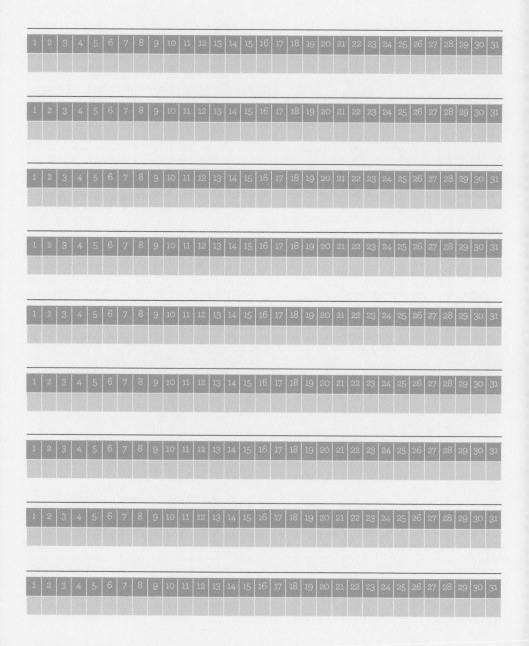

Weight

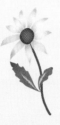

Month:

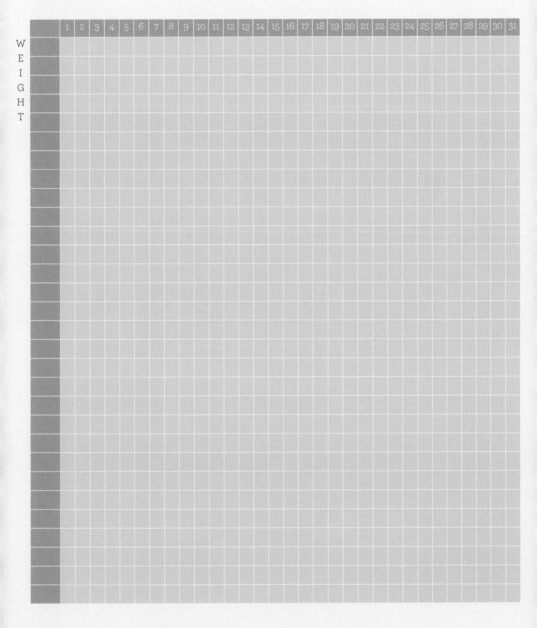

WEIGHT

	1	2	3	4	5	6	7	8	9	10	11	12	13	14	15	16	17	18	19	20	21	22	23	24	25	26	27	28	29	30	31

Cycle tracking

Month:

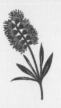

TEMPERATURE	1	2	3	4	5	6	7	8	9	10	11	12	13	14
37.30°C/99.4°F														
37.25°C/99.3°F														
37.20°C/99.2°F														
37.15°C/99.1°F														
37.10°C/99.0°F														
37.05°C/98.9°F														
37.00°C/98.8°F														
36.95°C/98.7°F														
36.90°C/98.6°F														
36.85°C/98.5°F														
36.80°C/98.4°F														
36.75°C/98.3°F														
36.70°C/98.2°F														
36.65°C/98.1°F														
36.60°C/98.0°F														
36.55°C/97.9°F														
36.50°C/97.8°F														
36.45°C/97.7°F														
36.40°C/97.6°F														
36.35°C/97.5°F														
36.30°C/97.4°F														
36.25°C/97.3°F														
36.20°C/97.2°F														
36.15°C/97.1°F														
36.10°C/97.0°F														
36.05°C/96.9°F														
36.00°C/96.8°F														
35.95°C/96.7°F														
35.90°C/96.6°F														

Cervical fluid														
Cervical position														
Cervical texture														
Sex														
Ovulation test														
Pregnancy test														
Period														
Day of cycle														

CERVICAL FLUID: **S** – Sticky   **C** – Creamy   **W** – Watery   **E** – Egg white

CERVICAL POSITION: **L** – Low   **M** – Medium   **H** – High

CERVICAL TEXTURE: **S** – Soft   **M** – Medium   **F** – Firm

15	16	17	18	19	20	21	22	23	24	25	26	27	28	29	30	31

Symptoms & treatments

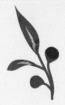

Month:

SYMPTOM:

	1	2	3	4	5	6	7	8	9	10	11	12	13	14	15	16	17	18	19	20	21	22	23	24	25	26	27	28	29	30	31
😀																															
🙂																															
😐																															
🙁																															
☹️																															

SYMPTOM:

	1	2	3	4	5	6	7	8	9	10	11	12	13	14	15	16	17	18	19	20	21	22	23	24	25	26	27	28	29	30	31
😀																															
🙂																															
😐																															
🙁																															
☹️																															

SYMPTOM:

	1	2	3	4	5	6	7	8	9	10	11	12	13	14	15	16	17	18	19	20	21	22	23	24	25	26	27	28	29	30	31
😀																															
🙂																															
😐																															
🙁																															
☹️																															

SYMPTOM:

	1	2	3	4	5	6	7	8	9	10	11	12	13	14	15	16	17	18	19	20	21	22	23	24	25	26	27	28	29	30	31
😀																															
🙂																															
😐																															
🙁																															
☹️																															

SYMPTOM:

	1	2	3	4	5	6	7	8	9	10	11	12	13	14	15	16	17	18	19	20	21	22	23	24	25	26	27	28	29	30	31
😀																															
🙂																															
😐																															
🙁																															
☹️																															

SYMPTOM:

	1	2	3	4	5	6	7	8	9	10	11	12	13	14	15	16	17	18	19	20	21	22	23	24	25	26	27	28	29	30	31
😄																															
🙂																															
😐																															
🙁																															
☹️																															

SYMPTOM:

	1	2	3	4	5	6	7	8	9	10	11	12	13	14	15	16	17	18	19	20	21	22	23	24	25	26	27	28	29	30	31
😄																															
🙂																															
😐																															
🙁																															
☹️																															

SYMPTOM:

	1	2	3	4	5	6	7	8	9	10	11	12	13	14	15	16	17	18	19	20	21	22	23	24	25	26	27	28	29	30	31
😄																															
🙂																															
😐																															
🙁																															
☹️																															

SYMPTOM:

	1	2	3	4	5	6	7	8	9	10	11	12	13	14	15	16	17	18	19	20	21	22	23	24	25	26	27	28	29	30	31
😄																															
🙂																															
😐																															
🙁																															
☹️																															

TREATMENT STARTED: A

B _____ C _____

D _____ E _____

F _____ G _____

	1	2	3	4	5	6	7	8	9	10	11	12	13	14	15	16	17	18	19	20	21	22	23	24	25	26	27	28	29	30	31
A																															
B																															
C																															
D																															
E																															
F																															
G																															

Habits

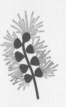

Month:

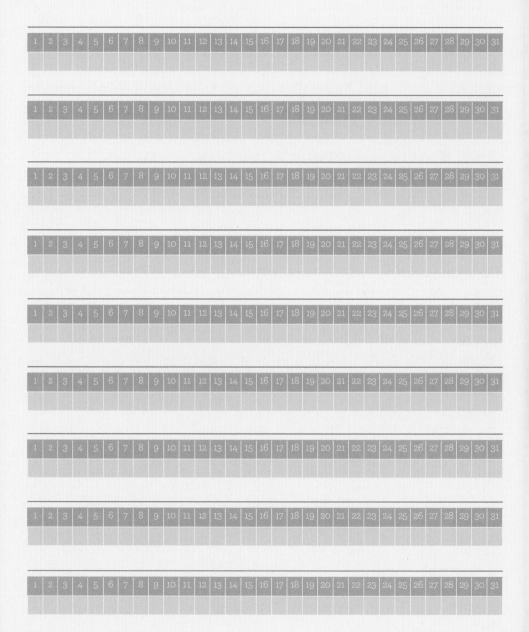

1	2	3	4	5	6	7	8	9	10	11	12	13	14	15	16	17	18	19	20	21	22	23	24	25	26	27	28	29	30	31

1	2	3	4	5	6	7	8	9	10	11	12	13	14	15	16	17	18	19	20	21	22	23	24	25	26	27	28	29	30	31

1	2	3	4	5	6	7	8	9	10	11	12	13	14	15	16	17	18	19	20	21	22	23	24	25	26	27	28	29	30	31

1	2	3	4	5	6	7	8	9	10	11	12	13	14	15	16	17	18	19	20	21	22	23	24	25	26	27	28	29	30	31

1	2	3	4	5	6	7	8	9	10	11	12	13	14	15	16	17	18	19	20	21	22	23	24	25	26	27	28	29	30	31

1	2	3	4	5	6	7	8	9	10	11	12	13	14	15	16	17	18	19	20	21	22	23	24	25	26	27	28	29	30	31

1	2	3	4	5	6	7	8	9	10	11	12	13	14	15	16	17	18	19	20	21	22	23	24	25	26	27	28	29	30	31

1	2	3	4	5	6	7	8	9	10	11	12	13	14	15	16	17	18	19	20	21	22	23	24	25	26	27	28	29	30	31

1	2	3	4	5	6	7	8	9	10	11	12	13	14	15	16	17	18	19	20	21	22	23	24	25	26	27	28	29	30	31

Weight

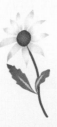

Month:

	1	2	3	4	5	6	7	8	9	10	11	12	13	14	15	16	17	18	19	20	21	22	23	24	25	26	27	28	29	30	31
W E I G H T																															

Cycle tracking

Month: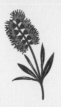

TEMPERATURE	1	2	3	4	5	6	7	8	9	10	11	12	13	14
37.30°C/99.4°F														
37.25°C/99.3°F														
37.20°C/99.2°F														
37.15°C/99.1°F														
37.10°C/99.0°F														
37.05°C/98.9°F														
37.00°C/98.8°F														
36.95°C/98.7°F														
36.90°C/98.6°F														
36.85°C/98.5°F														
36.80°C/98.4°F														
36.75°C/98.3°F														
36.70°C/98.2°F														
36.65°C/98.1°F														
36.60°C/98.0°F														
36.55°C/97.9°F														
36.50°C/97.8°F														
36.45°C/97.7°F														
36.40°C/97.6°F														
36.35°C/97.5°F														
36.30°C/97.4°F														
36.25°C/97.3°F														
36.20°C/97.2°F														
36.15°C/97.1°F														
36.10°C/97.0°F														
36.05°C/96.9°F														
36.00°C/96.8°F														
35.95°C/96.7°F														
35.90°C/96.6°F														

Cervical fluid														
Cervical position														
Cervical texture														
Sex														
Ovulation test														
Pregnancy test														
Period														
Day of cycle														

CERVICAL FLUID: **S** – Sticky   **C** – Creamy   **W** – Watery   **E** – Egg white

CERVICAL POSITION: **L** – Low   **M** – Medium   **H** – High

CERVICAL TEXTURE: **S** – Soft   **M** – Medium   **F** – Firm

15	16	17	18	19	20	21	22	23	24	25	26	27	28	29	30	31

Symptoms & treatments

Month:

SYMPTOM:

	1	2	3	4	5	6	7	8	9	10	11	12	13	14	15	16	17	18	19	20	21	22	23	24	25	26	27	28	29	30	31
😄																															
🙂																															
😐																															
🙁																															
😞																															

SYMPTOM:

	1	2	3	4	5	6	7	8	9	10	11	12	13	14	15	16	17	18	19	20	21	22	23	24	25	26	27	28	29	30	31
😄																															
🙂																															
😐																															
🙁																															
😞																															

SYMPTOM:

	1	2	3	4	5	6	7	8	9	10	11	12	13	14	15	16	17	18	19	20	21	22	23	24	25	26	27	28	29	30	31
😄																															
🙂																															
😐																															
🙁																															
😞																															

SYMPTOM:

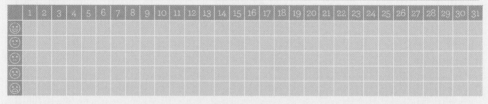

	1	2	3	4	5	6	7	8	9	10	11	12	13	14	15	16	17	18	19	20	21	22	23	24	25	26	27	28	29	30	31
😄																															
🙂																															
😐																															
🙁																															
😞																															

SYMPTOM:

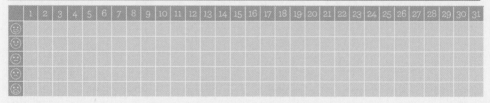

	1	2	3	4	5	6	7	8	9	10	11	12	13	14	15	16	17	18	19	20	21	22	23	24	25	26	27	28	29	30	31
😄																															
🙂																															
😐																															
🙁																															
😞																															

SYMPTOM:

	1	2	3	4	5	6	7	8	9	10	11	12	13	14	15	16	17	18	19	20	21	22	23	24	25	26	27	28	29	30	31
😀																															
🙂																															
😐																															
🙁																															
😟																															

SYMPTOM:

	1	2	3	4	5	6	7	8	9	10	11	12	13	14	15	16	17	18	19	20	21	22	23	24	25	26	27	28	29	30	31
😀																															
🙂																															
😐																															
🙁																															
😟																															

SYMPTOM:

	1	2	3	4	5	6	7	8	9	10	11	12	13	14	15	16	17	18	19	20	21	22	23	24	25	26	27	28	29	30	31
😀																															
🙂																															
😐																															
🙁																															
😟																															

SYMPTOM:

	1	2	3	4	5	6	7	8	9	10	11	12	13	14	15	16	17	18	19	20	21	22	23	24	25	26	27	28	29	30	31
😀																															
🙂																															
😐																															
🙁																															
😟																															

TREATMENT STARTED: **A**

B   C

D   E

F   G

	1	2	3	4	5	6	7	8	9	10	11	12	13	14	15	16	17	18	19	20	21	22	23	24	25	26	27	28	29	30	31
A																															
B																															
C																															
D																															
E																															
F																															
G																															

Habits

Month:

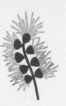

1	2	3	4	5	6	7	8	9	10	11	12	13	14	15	16	17	18	19	20	21	22	23	24	25	26	27	28	29	30	31

1	2	3	4	5	6	7	8	9	10	11	12	13	14	15	16	17	18	19	20	21	22	23	24	25	26	27	28	29	30	31

1	2	3	4	5	6	7	8	9	10	11	12	13	14	15	16	17	18	19	20	21	22	23	24	25	26	27	28	29	30	31

1	2	3	4	5	6	7	8	9	10	11	12	13	14	15	16	17	18	19	20	21	22	23	24	25	26	27	28	29	30	31

1	2	3	4	5	6	7	8	9	10	11	12	13	14	15	16	17	18	19	20	21	22	23	24	25	26	27	28	29	30	31

1	2	3	4	5	6	7	8	9	10	11	12	13	14	15	16	17	18	19	20	21	22	23	24	25	26	27	28	29	30	31

1	2	3	4	5	6	7	8	9	10	11	12	13	14	15	16	17	18	19	20	21	22	23	24	25	26	27	28	29	30	31

1	2	3	4	5	6	7	8	9	10	11	12	13	14	15	16	17	18	19	20	21	22	23	24	25	26	27	28	29	30	31

Weight

Month:

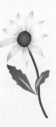

	1	2	3	4	5	6	7	8	9	10	11	12	13	14	15	16	17	18	19	20	21	22	23	24	25	26	27	28	29	30	31
W E I G H T																															

Cycle tracking

Month: _____

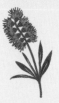

TEMPERATURE	1	2	3	4	5	6	7	8	9	10	11	12	13	14
37.30°C/99.4°F														
37.25°C/99.3°F														
37.20°C/99.2°F														
37.15°C/99.1°F														
37.10°C/99.0°F														
37.05°C/98.9°F														
37.00°C/98.8°F														
36.95°C/98.7°F														
36.90°C/98.6°F														
36.85°C/98.5°F														
36.80°C/98.4°F														
36.75°C/98.3°F														
36.70°C/98.2°F														
36.65°C/98.1°F														
36.60°C/98.0°F														
36.55°C/97.9°F														
36.50°C/97.8°F														
36.45°C/97.7°F														
36.40°C/97.6°F														
36.35°C/97.5°F														
36.30°C/97.4°F														
36.25°C/97.3°F														
36.20°C/97.2°F														
36.15°C/97.1°F														
36.10°C/97.0°F														
36.05°C/96.9°F														
36.00°C/96.8°F														
35.95°C/96.7°F														
35.90°C/96.6°F														

Cervical fluid														
Cervical position														
Cervical texture														
Sex														
Ovulation test														
Pregnancy test														
Period														
Day of cycle														

CERVICAL FLUID: **S** – Sticky   **C** – Creamy   **W** – Watery   **E** – Egg white

CERVICAL POSITION: **L** – Low   **M** – Medium   **H** – High

CERVICAL TEXTURE: **S** – Soft   **M** – Medium   **F** – Firm

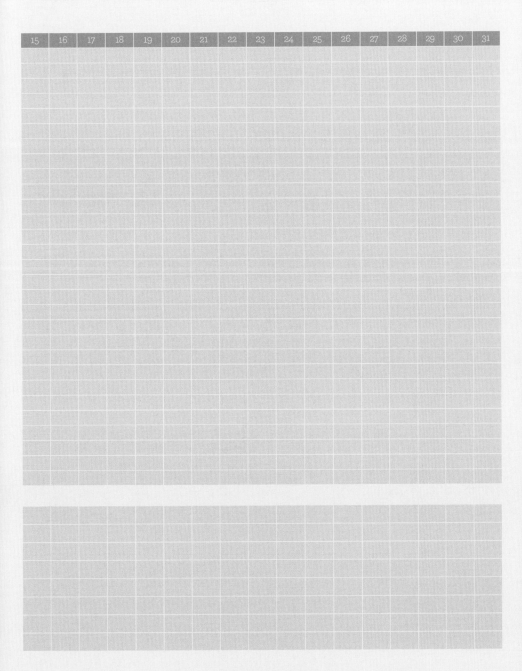

15	16	17	18	19	20	21	22	23	24	25	26	27	28	29	30	31

Symptoms & treatments

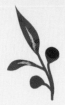

Month:

SYMPTOM:

	1	2	3	4	5	6	7	8	9	10	11	12	13	14	15	16	17	18	19	20	21	22	23	24	25	26	27	28	29	30	31
😄																															
🙂																															
😐																															
🙁																															
😣																															

SYMPTOM:

	1	2	3	4	5	6	7	8	9	10	11	12	13	14	15	16	17	18	19	20	21	22	23	24	25	26	27	28	29	30	31
😄																															
🙂																															
😐																															
🙁																															
😣																															

SYMPTOM:

	1	2	3	4	5	6	7	8	9	10	11	12	13	14	15	16	17	18	19	20	21	22	23	24	25	26	27	28	29	30	31
😄																															
🙂																															
😐																															
🙁																															
😣																															

SYMPTOM:

	1	2	3	4	5	6	7	8	9	10	11	12	13	14	15	16	17	18	19	20	21	22	23	24	25	26	27	28	29	30	31
😄																															
🙂																															
😐																															
🙁																															
😣																															

SYMPTOM:

	1	2	3	4	5	6	7	8	9	10	11	12	13	14	15	16	17	18	19	20	21	22	23	24	25	26	27	28	29	30	31
😄																															
🙂																															
😐																															
🙁																															
😣																															

SYMPTOM: _____

	1	2	3	4	5	6	7	8	9	10	11	12	13	14	15	16	17	18	19	20	21	22	23	24	25	26	27	28	29	30	31
☺																															
☺																															
☺																															
☹																															
☹																															

SYMPTOM: _____

	1	2	3	4	5	6	7	8	9	10	11	12	13	14	15	16	17	18	19	20	21	22	23	24	25	26	27	28	29	30	31
☺																															
☺																															
☺																															
☹																															
☹																															

SYMPTOM: _____

	1	2	3	4	5	6	7	8	9	10	11	12	13	14	15	16	17	18	19	20	21	22	23	24	25	26	27	28	29	30	31
☺																															
☺																															
☺																															
☹																															
☹																															

SYMPTOM: _____

	1	2	3	4	5	6	7	8	9	10	11	12	13	14	15	16	17	18	19	20	21	22	23	24	25	26	27	28	29	30	31
☺																															
☺																															
☺																															
☹																															
☹																															

TREATMENT STARTED: **A**

B _____   C _____

D _____   E _____

F _____   G _____

	1	2	3	4	5	6	7	8	9	10	11	12	13	14	15	16	17	18	19	20	21	22	23	24	25	26	27	28	29	30	31
A																															
B																															
C																															
D																															
E																															
F																															
G																															

Habits

Month:

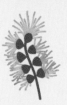

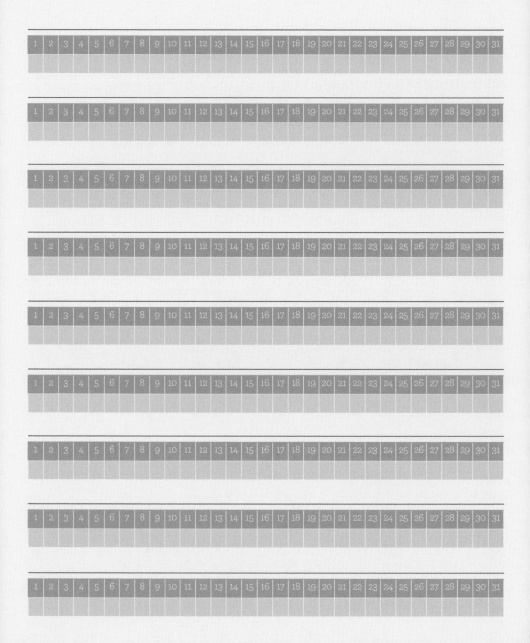

1	2	3	4	5	6	7	8	9	10	11	12	13	14	15	16	17	18	19	20	21	22	23	24	25	26	27	28	29	30	31

1	2	3	4	5	6	7	8	9	10	11	12	13	14	15	16	17	18	19	20	21	22	23	24	25	26	27	28	29	30	31

1	2	3	4	5	6	7	8	9	10	11	12	13	14	15	16	17	18	19	20	21	22	23	24	25	26	27	28	29	30	31

1	2	3	4	5	6	7	8	9	10	11	12	13	14	15	16	17	18	19	20	21	22	23	24	25	26	27	28	29	30	31

1	2	3	4	5	6	7	8	9	10	11	12	13	14	15	16	17	18	19	20	21	22	23	24	25	26	27	28	29	30	31

1	2	3	4	5	6	7	8	9	10	11	12	13	14	15	16	17	18	19	20	21	22	23	24	25	26	27	28	29	30	31

1	2	3	4	5	6	7	8	9	10	11	12	13	14	15	16	17	18	19	20	21	22	23	24	25	26	27	28	29	30	31

1	2	3	4	5	6	7	8	9	10	11	12	13	14	15	16	17	18	19	20	21	22	23	24	25	26	27	28	29	30	31

Weight

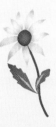

Month:

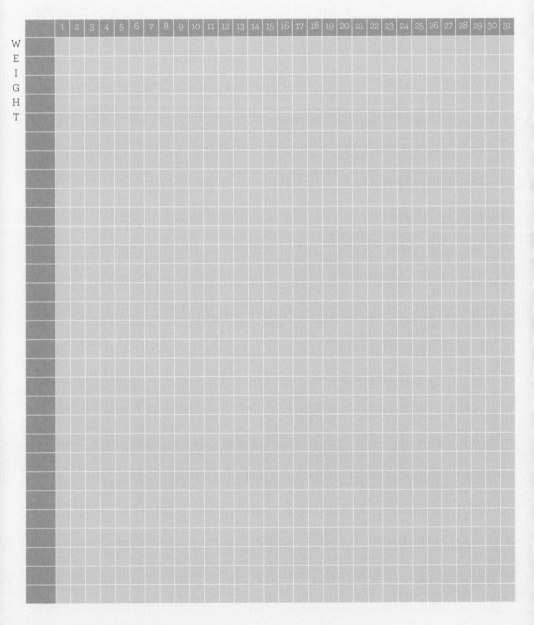

W
E
I
G
H
T

	1	2	3	4	5	6	7	8	9	10	11	12	13	14	15	16	17	18	19	20	21	22	23	24	25	26	27	28	29	30	31

Cycle tracking

Month:

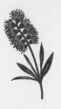

TEMPERATURE	1	2	3	4	5	6	7	8	9	10	11	12	13	14
37.30°C/99.4°F														
37.25°C/99.3°F														
37.20°C/99.2°F														
37.15°C/99.1°F														
37.10°C/99.0°F														
37.05°C/98.9°F														
37.00°C/98.8°F														
36.95°C/98.7°F														
36.90°C/98.6°F														
36.85°C/98.5°F														
36.80°C/98.4°F														
36.75°C/98.3°F														
36.70°C/98.2°F														
36.65°C/98.1°F														
36.60°C/98.0°F														
36.55°C/97.9°F														
36.50°C/97.8°F														
36.45°C/97.7°F														
36.40°C/97.6°F														
36.35°C/97.5°F														
36.30°C/97.4°F														
36.25°C/97.3°F														
36.20°C/97.2°F														
36.15°C/97.1°F														
36.10°C/97.0°F														
36.05°C/96.9°F														
36.00°C/96.8°F														
35.95°C/96.7°F														
35.90°C/96.6°F														

Cervical fluid														
Cervical position														
Cervical texture														
Sex														
Ovulation test														
Pregnancy test														
Period														
Day of cycle														

CERVICAL FLUID: **S** – Sticky   **C** – Creamy   **W** – Watery   **E** – Egg white

CERVICAL POSITION: **L** – Low   **M** – Medium   **H** – High

CERVICAL TEXTURE: **S** – Soft   **M** – Medium   **F** – Firm

15	16	17	18	19	20	21	22	23	24	25	26	27	28	29	30	31

Symptoms & treatments

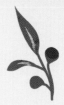

SYMPTOM:

	1	2	3	4	5	6	7	8	9	10	11	12	13	14	15	16	17	18	19	20	21	22	23	24	25	26	27	28	29	30	31
😄																															
🙂																															
😐																															
🙁																															
☹️																															

SYMPTOM:

	1	2	3	4	5	6	7	8	9	10	11	12	13	14	15	16	17	18	19	20	21	22	23	24	25	26	27	28	29	30	31
😄																															
🙂																															
😐																															
🙁																															
☹️																															

SYMPTOM:

	1	2	3	4	5	6	7	8	9	10	11	12	13	14	15	16	17	18	19	20	21	22	23	24	25	26	27	28	29	30	31
😄																															
🙂																															
😐																															
🙁																															
☹️																															

SYMPTOM:

	1	2	3	4	5	6	7	8	9	10	11	12	13	14	15	16	17	18	19	20	21	22	23	24	25	26	27	28	29	30	31
😄																															
🙂																															
😐																															
🙁																															
☹️																															

SYMPTOM:

	1	2	3	4	5	6	7	8	9	10	11	12	13	14	15	16	17	18	19	20	21	22	23	24	25	26	27	28	29	30	31
😄																															
🙂																															
😐																															
🙁																															
☹️																															

SYMPTOM:

	1	2	3	4	5	6	7	8	9	10	11	12	13	14	15	16	17	18	19	20	21	22	23	24	25	26	27	28	29	30	31
☺																															
☺																															
☺																															
☹																															
☹																															

SYMPTOM:

	1	2	3	4	5	6	7	8	9	10	11	12	13	14	15	16	17	18	19	20	21	22	23	24	25	26	27	28	29	30	31
☺																															
☺																															
☺																															
☹																															
☹																															

SYMPTOM:

	1	2	3	4	5	6	7	8	9	10	11	12	13	14	15	16	17	18	19	20	21	22	23	24	25	26	27	28	29	30	31
☺																															
☺																															
☺																															
☹																															
☹																															

SYMPTOM:

	1	2	3	4	5	6	7	8	9	10	11	12	13	14	15	16	17	18	19	20	21	22	23	24	25	26	27	28	29	30	31
☺																															
☺																															
☺																															
☹																															
☹																															

TREATMENT STARTED: **A**

B   C

D   E

F   G

	1	2	3	4	5	6	7	8	9	10	11	12	13	14	15	16	17	18	19	20	21	22	23	24	25	26	27	28	29	30	31
A																															
B																															
C																															
D																															
E																															
F																															
G																															

Habits

Month:

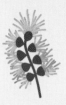

1	2	3	4	5	6	7	8	9	10	11	12	13	14	15	16	17	18	19	20	21	22	23	24	25	26	27	28	29	30	31

1	2	3	4	5	6	7	8	9	10	11	12	13	14	15	16	17	18	19	20	21	22	23	24	25	26	27	28	29	30	31

1	2	3	4	5	6	7	8	9	10	11	12	13	14	15	16	17	18	19	20	21	22	23	24	25	26	27	28	29	30	31

1	2	3	4	5	6	7	8	9	10	11	12	13	14	15	16	17	18	19	20	21	22	23	24	25	26	27	28	29	30	31

1	2	3	4	5	6	7	8	9	10	11	12	13	14	15	16	17	18	19	20	21	22	23	24	25	26	27	28	29	30	31

1	2	3	4	5	6	7	8	9	10	11	12	13	14	15	16	17	18	19	20	21	22	23	24	25	26	27	28	29	30	31

1	2	3	4	5	6	7	8	9	10	11	12	13	14	15	16	17	18	19	20	21	22	23	24	25	26	27	28	29	30	31

1	2	3	4	5	6	7	8	9	10	11	12	13	14	15	16	17	18	19	20	21	22	23	24	25	26	27	28	29	30	31

1	2	3	4	5	6	7	8	9	10	11	12	13	14	15	16	17	18	19	20	21	22	23	24	25	26	27	28	29	30	31

Weight

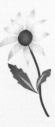

Month:

	1	2	3	4	5	6	7	8	9	10	11	12	13	14	15	16	17	18	19	20	21	22	23	24	25	26	27	28	29	30	31
W																															
E																															
I																															
G																															
H																															
T																															

Cycle tracking

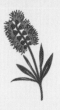

Month:

TEMPERATURE	1	2	3	4	5	6	7	8	9	10	11	12	13	14
37.30°C/99.4°F														
37.25°C/99.3°F														
37.20°C/99.2°F														
37.15°C/99.1°F														
37.10°C/99.0°F														
37.05°C/98.9°F														
37.00°C/98.8°F														
36.95°C/98.7°F														
36.90°C/98.6°F														
36.85°C/98.5°F														
36.80°C/98.4°F														
36.75°C/98.3°F														
36.70°C/98.2°F														
36.65°C/98.1°F														
36.60°C/98.0°F														
36.55°C/97.9°F														
36.50°C/97.8°F														
36.45°C/97.7°F														
36.40°C/97.6°F														
36.35°C/97.5°F														
36.30°C/97.4°F														
36.25°C/97.3°F														
36.20°C/97.2°F														
36.15°C/97.1°F														
36.10°C/97.0°F														
36.05°C/96.9°F														
36.00°C/96.8°F														
35.95°C/96.7°F														
35.90°C/96.6°F														

Cervical fluid														
Cervical position														
Cervical texture														
Sex														
Ovulation test														
Pregnancy test														
Period														
Day of cycle														

CERVICAL FLUID: **S** – Sticky   **C** – Creamy   **W** – Watery   **E** – Egg white

CERVICAL POSITION: **L** – Low   **M** – Medium   **H** – High

CERVICAL TEXTURE: **S** – Soft   **M** – Medium   **F** – Firm

15	16	17	18	19	20	21	22	23	24	25	26	27	28	29	30	31

Symptoms & treatments

Month:

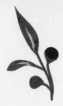

SYMPTOM:

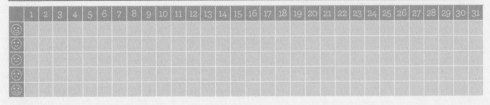

| | 1 | 2 | 3 | 4 | 5 | 6 | 7 | 8 | 9 | 10 | 11 | 12 | 13 | 14 | 15 | 16 | 17 | 18 | 19 | 20 | 21 | 22 | 23 | 24 | 25 | 26 | 27 | 28 | 29 | 30 | 31 |

SYMPTOM:

| | 1 | 2 | 3 | 4 | 5 | 6 | 7 | 8 | 9 | 10 | 11 | 12 | 13 | 14 | 15 | 16 | 17 | 18 | 19 | 20 | 21 | 22 | 23 | 24 | 25 | 26 | 27 | 28 | 29 | 30 | 31 |

SYMPTOM:

| | 1 | 2 | 3 | 4 | 5 | 6 | 7 | 8 | 9 | 10 | 11 | 12 | 13 | 14 | 15 | 16 | 17 | 18 | 19 | 20 | 21 | 22 | 23 | 24 | 25 | 26 | 27 | 28 | 29 | 30 | 31 |

SYMPTOM:

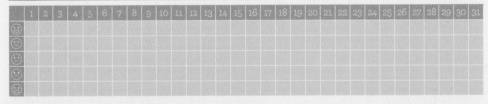

| | 1 | 2 | 3 | 4 | 5 | 6 | 7 | 8 | 9 | 10 | 11 | 12 | 13 | 14 | 15 | 16 | 17 | 18 | 19 | 20 | 21 | 22 | 23 | 24 | 25 | 26 | 27 | 28 | 29 | 30 | 31 |

SYMPTOM:

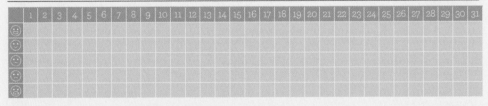

| | 1 | 2 | 3 | 4 | 5 | 6 | 7 | 8 | 9 | 10 | 11 | 12 | 13 | 14 | 15 | 16 | 17 | 18 | 19 | 20 | 21 | 22 | 23 | 24 | 25 | 26 | 27 | 28 | 29 | 30 | 31 |

SYMPTOM:

	1	2	3	4	5	6	7	8	9	10	11	12	13	14	15	16	17	18	19	20	21	22	23	24	25	26	27	28	29	30	31
😀																															
🙂																															
😐																															
🙁																															
😞																															

SYMPTOM:

	1	2	3	4	5	6	7	8	9	10	11	12	13	14	15	16	17	18	19	20	21	22	23	24	25	26	27	28	29	30	31
😀																															
🙂																															
😐																															
🙁																															
😞																															

SYMPTOM:

	1	2	3	4	5	6	7	8	9	10	11	12	13	14	15	16	17	18	19	20	21	22	23	24	25	26	27	28	29	30	31
😀																															
🙂																															
😐																															
🙁																															
😞																															

SYMPTOM:

	1	2	3	4	5	6	7	8	9	10	11	12	13	14	15	16	17	18	19	20	21	22	23	24	25	26	27	28	29	30	31
😀																															
🙂																															
😐																															
🙁																															
😞																															

TREATMENT STARTED: A

B

C

D

E

F

G

	1	2	3	4	5	6	7	8	9	10	11	12	13	14	15	16	17	18	19	20	21	22	23	24	25	26	27	28	29	30	31
A																															
B																															
C																															
D																															
E																															
F																															
G																															

Habits

Month:

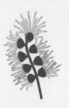

1	2	3	4	5	6	7	8	9	10	11	12	13	14	15	16	17	18	19	20	21	22	23	24	25	26	27	28	29	30	31

1	2	3	4	5	6	7	8	9	10	11	12	13	14	15	16	17	18	19	20	21	22	23	24	25	26	27	28	29	30	31

1	2	3	4	5	6	7	8	9	10	11	12	13	14	15	16	17	18	19	20	21	22	23	24	25	26	27	28	29	30	31

1	2	3	4	5	6	7	8	9	10	11	12	13	14	15	16	17	18	19	20	21	22	23	24	25	26	27	28	29	30	31

1	2	3	4	5	6	7	8	9	10	11	12	13	14	15	16	17	18	19	20	21	22	23	24	25	26	27	28	29	30	31

1	2	3	4	5	6	7	8	9	10	11	12	13	14	15	16	17	18	19	20	21	22	23	24	25	26	27	28	29	30	31

1	2	3	4	5	6	7	8	9	10	11	12	13	14	15	16	17	18	19	20	21	22	23	24	25	26	27	28	29	30	31

1	2	3	4	5	6	7	8	9	10	11	12	13	14	15	16	17	18	19	20	21	22	23	24	25	26	27	28	29	30	31

1	2	3	4	5	6	7	8	9	10	11	12	13	14	15	16	17	18	19	20	21	22	23	24	25	26	27	28	29	30	31

Weight

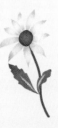

Month:

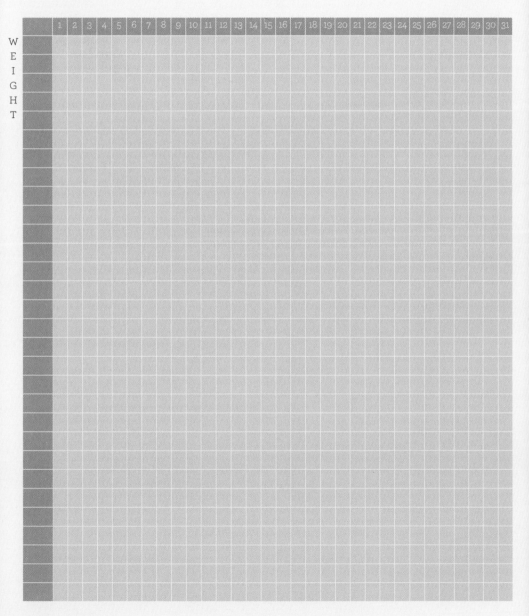

W E I G H T

	1	2	3	4	5	6	7	8	9	10	11	12	13	14	15	16	17	18	19	20	21	22	23	24	25	26	27	28	29	30	31

Cycle tracking

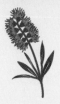

Month:

TEMPERATURE	1	2	3	4	5	6	7	8	9	10	11	12	13	14
37.30°C/99.4°F														
37.25°C/99.3°F														
37.20°C/99.2°F														
37.15°C/99.1°F														
37.10°C/99.0°F														
37.05°C/98.9°F														
37.00°C/98.8°F														
36.95°C/98.7°F														
36.90°C/98.6°F														
36.85°C/98.5°F														
36.80°C/98.4°F														
36.75°C/98.3°F														
36.70°C/98.2°F														
36.65°C/98.1°F														
36.60°C/98.0°F														
36.55°C/97.9°F														
36.50°C/97.8°F														
36.45°C/97.7°F														
36.40°C/97.6°F														
36.35°C/97.5°F														
36.30°C/97.4°F														
36.25°C/97.3°F														
36.20°C/97.2°F														
36.15°C/97.1°F														
36.10°C/97.0°F														
36.05°C/96.9°F														
36.00°C/96.8°F														
35.95°C/96.7°F														
35.90°C/96.6°F														

Cervical fluid														
Cervical position														
Cervical texture														
Sex														
Ovulation test														
Pregnancy test														
Period														
Day of cycle														

CERVICAL FLUID: **S** – Sticky   **C** – Creamy   **W** – Watery   **E** – Egg white

CERVICAL POSITION: **L** – Low   **M** – Medium   **H** – High

CERVICAL TEXTURE: **S** – Soft   **M** – Medium   **F** – Firm

15	16	17	18	19	20	21	22	23	24	25	26	27	28	29	30	31

Symptoms & treatments

Month:

SYMPTOM:

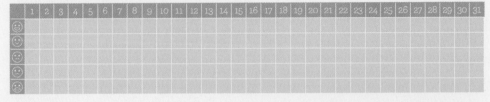

SYMPTOM:

	1	2	3	4	5	6	7	8	9	10	11	12	13	14	15	16	17	18	19	20	21	22	23	24	25	26	27	28	29	30	31

SYMPTOM:

	1	2	3	4	5	6	7	8	9	10	11	12	13	14	15	16	17	18	19	20	21	22	23	24	25	26	27	28	29	30	31

SYMPTOM:

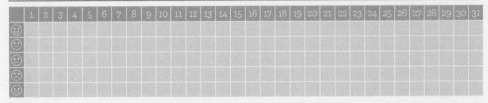

SYMPTOM:

	1	2	3	4	5	6	7	8	9	10	11	12	13	14	15	16	17	18	19	20	21	22	23	24	25	26	27	28	29	30	31

SYMPTOM:

	1	2	3	4	5	6	7	8	9	10	11	12	13	14	15	16	17	18	19	20	21	22	23	24	25	26	27	28	29	30	31
😊																															
🙂																															
😐																															
🙁																															
☹️																															

SYMPTOM:

	1	2	3	4	5	6	7	8	9	10	11	12	13	14	15	16	17	18	19	20	21	22	23	24	25	26	27	28	29	30	31
😊																															
🙂																															
😐																															
🙁																															
☹️																															

SYMPTOM:

	1	2	3	4	5	6	7	8	9	10	11	12	13	14	15	16	17	18	19	20	21	22	23	24	25	26	27	28	29	30	31
😊																															
🙂																															
😐																															
🙁																															
☹️																															

SYMPTOM:

	1	2	3	4	5	6	7	8	9	10	11	12	13	14	15	16	17	18	19	20	21	22	23	24	25	26	27	28	29	30	31
😊																															
🙂																															
😐																															
🙁																															
☹️																															

TREATMENT STARTED: **A**

B   C

D   E

F   G

	1	2	3	4	5	6	7	8	9	10	11	12	13	14	15	16	17	18	19	20	21	22	23	24	25	26	27	28	29	30	31
A																															
B																															
C																															
D																															
E																															
F																															
G																															

Habits

Month:

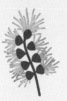

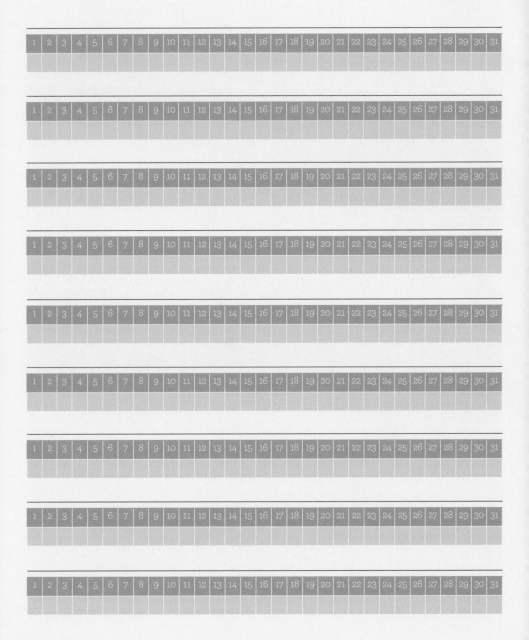

1	2	3	4	5	6	7	8	9	10	11	12	13	14	15	16	17	18	19	20	21	22	23	24	25	26	27	28	29	30	31

1	2	3	4	5	6	7	8	9	10	11	12	13	14	15	16	17	18	19	20	21	22	23	24	25	26	27	28	29	30	31

1	2	3	4	5	6	7	8	9	10	11	12	13	14	15	16	17	18	19	20	21	22	23	24	25	26	27	28	29	30	31

1	2	3	4	5	6	7	8	9	10	11	12	13	14	15	16	17	18	19	20	21	22	23	24	25	26	27	28	29	30	31

1	2	3	4	5	6	7	8	9	10	11	12	13	14	15	16	17	18	19	20	21	22	23	24	25	26	27	28	29	30	31

1	2	3	4	5	6	7	8	9	10	11	12	13	14	15	16	17	18	19	20	21	22	23	24	25	26	27	28	29	30	31

1	2	3	4	5	6	7	8	9	10	11	12	13	14	15	16	17	18	19	20	21	22	23	24	25	26	27	28	29	30	31

1	2	3	4	5	6	7	8	9	10	11	12	13	14	15	16	17	18	19	20	21	22	23	24	25	26	27	28	29	30	31

1	2	3	4	5	6	7	8	9	10	11	12	13	14	15	16	17	18	19	20	21	22	23	24	25	26	27	28	29	30	31

Weight

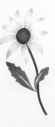

Month:

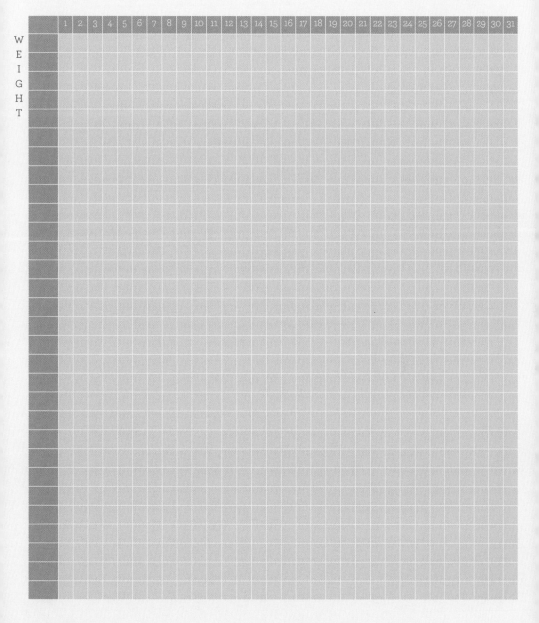

	1	2	3	4	5	6	7	8	9	10	11	12	13	14	15	16	17	18	19	20	21	22	23	24	25	26	27	28	29	30	31

W
E
I
G
H
T

Cycle tracking

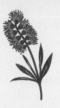

Month:

TEMPERATURE	1	2	3	4	5	6	7	8	9	10	11	12	13	14
37.30°C/99.4°F														
37.25°C/99.3°F														
37.20°C/99.2°F														
37.15°C/99.1°F														
37.10°C/99.0°F														
37.05°C/98.9°F														
37.00°C/98.8°F														
36.95°C/98.7°F														
36.90°C/98.6°F														
36.85°C/98.5°F														
36.80°C/98.4°F														
36.75°C/98.3°F														
36.70°C/98.2°F														
36.65°C/98.1°F														
36.60°C/98.0°F														
36.55°C/97.9°F														
36.50°C/97.8°F														
36.45°C/97.7°F														
36.40°C/97.6°F														
36.35°C/97.5°F														
36.30°C/97.4°F														
36.25°C/97.3°F														
36.20°C/97.2°F														
36.15°C/97.1°F														
36.10°C/97.0°F														
36.05°C/96.9°F														
36.00°C/96.8°F														
35.95°C/96.7°F														
35.90°C/96.6°F														

Cervical fluid														
Cervical position														
Cervical texture														
Sex														
Ovulation test														
Pregnancy test														
Period														
Day of cycle														

CERVICAL FLUID: **S** – Sticky   **C** – Creamy   **W** – Watery   **E** – Egg white

CERVICAL POSITION: **L** – Low   **M** – Medium   **H** – High

CERVICAL TEXTURE: **S** – Soft   **M** – Medium   **F** – Firm

15	16	17	18	19	20	21	22	23	24	25	26	27	28	29	30	31

Symptoms & treatments

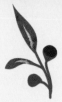

Month:

SYMPTOM:

	1	2	3	4	5	6	7	8	9	10	11	12	13	14	15	16	17	18	19	20	21	22	23	24	25	26	27	28	29	30	31
☺																															
☺																															
☺																															
☺																															
☹																															

SYMPTOM:

	1	2	3	4	5	6	7	8	9	10	11	12	13	14	15	16	17	18	19	20	21	22	23	24	25	26	27	28	29	30	31
☺																															
☺																															
☺																															
☺																															
☹																															

SYMPTOM:

	1	2	3	4	5	6	7	8	9	10	11	12	13	14	15	16	17	18	19	20	21	22	23	24	25	26	27	28	29	30	31
☺																															
☺																															
☺																															
☺																															
☹																															

SYMPTOM:

	1	2	3	4	5	6	7	8	9	10	11	12	13	14	15	16	17	18	19	20	21	22	23	24	25	26	27	28	29	30	31
☺																															
☺																															
☺																															
☺																															
☹																															

SYMPTOM:

	1	2	3	4	5	6	7	8	9	10	11	12	13	14	15	16	17	18	19	20	21	22	23	24	25	26	27	28	29	30	31
☺																															
☺																															
☺																															
☺																															
☹																															

SYMPTOM:

	1	2	3	4	5	6	7	8	9	10	11	12	13	14	15	16	17	18	19	20	21	22	23	24	25	26	27	28	29	30	31
☺																															
☺																															
☺																															
☹																															
☹																															

SYMPTOM:

	1	2	3	4	5	6	7	8	9	10	11	12	13	14	15	16	17	18	19	20	21	22	23	24	25	26	27	28	29	30	31
☺																															
☺																															
☺																															
☹																															
☹																															

SYMPTOM:

	1	2	3	4	5	6	7	8	9	10	11	12	13	14	15	16	17	18	19	20	21	22	23	24	25	26	27	28	29	30	31
☺																															
☺																															
☺																															
☹																															
☹																															

SYMPTOM:

	1	2	3	4	5	6	7	8	9	10	11	12	13	14	15	16	17	18	19	20	21	22	23	24	25	26	27	28	29	30	31
☺																															
☺																															
☺																															
☹																															
☹																															

TREATMENT STARTED: **A**

B   C

D   E

F   G

	1	2	3	4	5	6	7	8	9	10	11	12	13	14	15	16	17	18	19	20	21	22	23	24	25	26	27	28	29	30	31
A																															
B																															
C																															
D																															
E																															
F																															
G																															

Habits

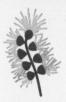

Month:

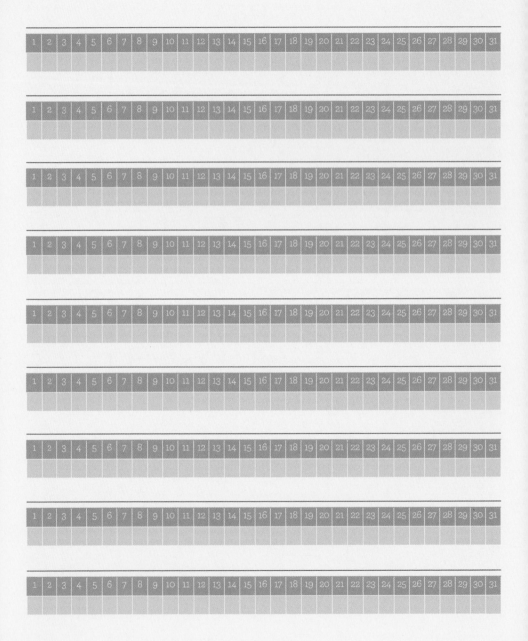

| 1 | 2 | 3 | 4 | 5 | 6 | 7 | 8 | 9 | 10 | 11 | 12 | 13 | 14 | 15 | 16 | 17 | 18 | 19 | 20 | 21 | 22 | 23 | 24 | 25 | 26 | 27 | 28 | 29 | 30 | 31 |

| 1 | 2 | 3 | 4 | 5 | 6 | 7 | 8 | 9 | 10 | 11 | 12 | 13 | 14 | 15 | 16 | 17 | 18 | 19 | 20 | 21 | 22 | 23 | 24 | 25 | 26 | 27 | 28 | 29 | 30 | 31 |

| 1 | 2 | 3 | 4 | 5 | 6 | 7 | 8 | 9 | 10 | 11 | 12 | 13 | 14 | 15 | 16 | 17 | 18 | 19 | 20 | 21 | 22 | 23 | 24 | 25 | 26 | 27 | 28 | 29 | 30 | 31 |

| 1 | 2 | 3 | 4 | 5 | 6 | 7 | 8 | 9 | 10 | 11 | 12 | 13 | 14 | 15 | 16 | 17 | 18 | 19 | 20 | 21 | 22 | 23 | 24 | 25 | 26 | 27 | 28 | 29 | 30 | 31 |

| 1 | 2 | 3 | 4 | 5 | 6 | 7 | 8 | 9 | 10 | 11 | 12 | 13 | 14 | 15 | 16 | 17 | 18 | 19 | 20 | 21 | 22 | 23 | 24 | 25 | 26 | 27 | 28 | 29 | 30 | 31 |

| 1 | 2 | 3 | 4 | 5 | 6 | 7 | 8 | 9 | 10 | 11 | 12 | 13 | 14 | 15 | 16 | 17 | 18 | 19 | 20 | 21 | 22 | 23 | 24 | 25 | 26 | 27 | 28 | 29 | 30 | 31 |

| 1 | 2 | 3 | 4 | 5 | 6 | 7 | 8 | 9 | 10 | 11 | 12 | 13 | 14 | 15 | 16 | 17 | 18 | 19 | 20 | 21 | 22 | 23 | 24 | 25 | 26 | 27 | 28 | 29 | 30 | 31 |

| 1 | 2 | 3 | 4 | 5 | 6 | 7 | 8 | 9 | 10 | 11 | 12 | 13 | 14 | 15 | 16 | 17 | 18 | 19 | 20 | 21 | 22 | 23 | 24 | 25 | 26 | 27 | 28 | 29 | 30 | 31 |

Weight

Month:

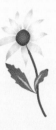

		1	2	3	4	5	6	7	8	9	10	11	12	13	14	15	16	17	18	19	20	21	22	23	24	25	26	27	28	29	30	31
W																																
E																																
I																																
G																																
H																																
T																																

Cycle tracking

Month:

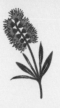

TEMPERATURE	1	2	3	4	5	6	7	8	9	10	11	12	13	14
37.30°C/99.4°F														
37.25°C/99.3°F														
37.20°C/99.2°F														
37.15°C/99.1°F														
37.10°C/99.0°F														
37.05°C/98.9°F														
37.00°C/98.8°F														
36.95°C/98.7°F														
36.90°C/98.6°F														
36.85°C/98.5°F														
36.80°C/98.4°F														
36.75°C/98.3°F														
36.70°C/98.2°F														
36.65°C/98.1°F														
36.60°C/98.0°F														
36.55°C/97.9°F														
36.50°C/97.8°F														
36.45°C/97.7°F														
36.40°C/97.6°F														
36.35°C/97.5°F														
36.30°C/97.4°F														
36.25°C/97.3°F														
36.20°C/97.2°F														
36.15°C/97.1°F														
36.10°C/97.0°F														
36.05°C/96.9°F														
36.00°C/96.8°F														
35.95°C/96.7°F														
35.90°C/96.6°F														

Cervical fluid														
Cervical position														
Cervical texture														
Sex														
Ovulation test														
Pregnancy test														
Period														
Day of cycle														

CERVICAL FLUID: **S** – Sticky   **C** – Creamy   **W** – Watery   **E** – Egg white

CERVICAL POSITION: **L** – Low   **M** – Medium   **H** – High

CERVICAL TEXTURE: **S** – Soft   **M** – Medium   **F** – Firm

15	16	17	18	19	20	21	22	23	24	25	26	27	28	29	30	31

Symptoms & treatments

Month:

SYMPTOM:

	1	2	3	4	5	6	7	8	9	10	11	12	13	14	15	16	17	18	19	20	21	22	23	24	25	26	27	28	29	30	31

SYMPTOM:

	1	2	3	4	5	6	7	8	9	10	11	12	13	14	15	16	17	18	19	20	21	22	23	24	25	26	27	28	29	30	31

SYMPTOM:

	1	2	3	4	5	6	7	8	9	10	11	12	13	14	15	16	17	18	19	20	21	22	23	24	25	26	27	28	29	30	31

SYMPTOM:

	1	2	3	4	5	6	7	8	9	10	11	12	13	14	15	16	17	18	19	20	21	22	23	24	25	26	27	28	29	30	31

SYMPTOM:

	1	2	3	4	5	6	7	8	9	10	11	12	13	14	15	16	17	18	19	20	21	22	23	24	25	26	27	28	29	30	31

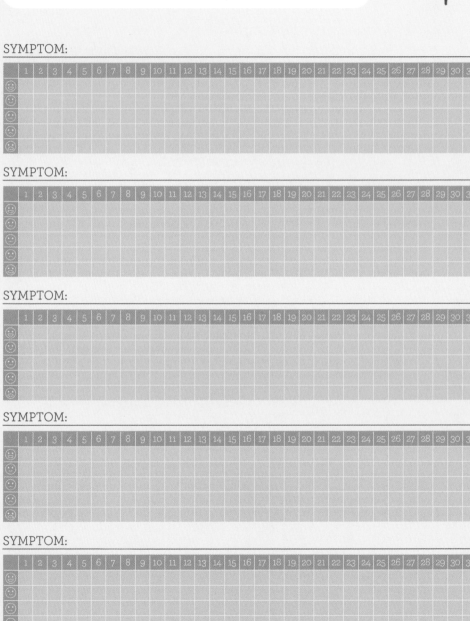

SYMPTOM: _____

	1	2	3	4	5	6	7	8	9	10	11	12	13	14	15	16	17	18	19	20	21	22	23	24	25	26	27	28	29	30	31
☺																															
☺																															
☺																															
☹																															
☹																															

SYMPTOM: _____

	1	2	3	4	5	6	7	8	9	10	11	12	13	14	15	16	17	18	19	20	21	22	23	24	25	26	27	28	29	30	31
☺																															
☺																															
☺																															
☹																															
☹																															

SYMPTOM: _____

	1	2	3	4	5	6	7	8	9	10	11	12	13	14	15	16	17	18	19	20	21	22	23	24	25	26	27	28	29	30	31
☺																															
☺																															
☺																															
☹																															
☹																															

SYMPTOM: _____

	1	2	3	4	5	6	7	8	9	10	11	12	13	14	15	16	17	18	19	20	21	22	23	24	25	26	27	28	29	30	31
☺																															
☺																															
☺																															
☹																															
☹																															

TREATMENT STARTED: **A** _____

B _____   C _____

D _____   E _____

F _____   G _____

	1	2	3	4	5	6	7	8	9	10	11	12	13	14	15	16	17	18	19	20	21	22	23	24	25	26	27	28	29	30	31
A																															
B																															
C																															
D																															
E																															
F																															
G																															

Habits

Month:

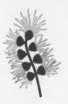

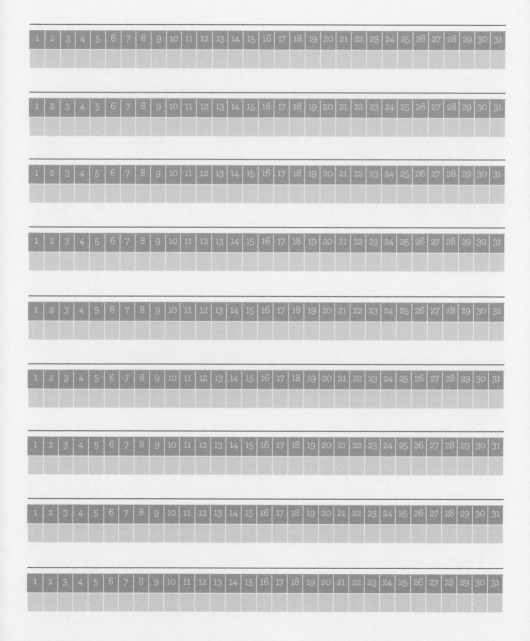

1	2	3	4	5	6	7	8	9	10	11	12	13	14	15	16	17	18	19	20	21	22	23	24	25	26	27	28	29	30	31

1	2	3	4	5	6	7	8	9	10	11	12	13	14	15	16	17	18	19	20	21	22	23	24	25	26	27	28	29	30	31

1	2	3	4	5	6	7	8	9	10	11	12	13	14	15	16	17	18	19	20	21	22	23	24	25	26	27	28	29	30	31

1	2	3	4	5	6	7	8	9	10	11	12	13	14	15	16	17	18	19	20	21	22	23	24	25	26	27	28	29	30	31

1	2	3	4	5	6	7	8	9	10	11	12	13	14	15	16	17	18	19	20	21	22	23	24	25	26	27	28	29	30	31

1	2	3	4	5	6	7	8	9	10	11	12	13	14	15	16	17	18	19	20	21	22	23	24	25	26	27	28	29	30	31

1	2	3	4	5	6	7	8	9	10	11	12	13	14	15	16	17	18	19	20	21	22	23	24	25	26	27	28	29	30	31

1	2	3	4	5	6	7	8	9	10	11	12	13	14	15	16	17	18	19	20	21	22	23	24	25	26	27	28	29	30	31

1	2	3	4	5	6	7	8	9	10	11	12	13	14	15	16	17	18	19	20	21	22	23	24	25	26	27	28	29	30	31

Weight

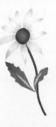

Month:

	1	2	3	4	5	6	7	8	9	10	11	12	13	14	15	16	17	18	19	20	21	22	23	24	25	26	27	28	29	30	31
W E I G H T																															

Cycle tracking

Month: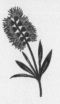

TEMPERATURE	1	2	3	4	5	6	7	8	9	10	11	12	13	14
37.30°C/99.4°F														
37.25°C/99.3°F														
37.20°C/99.2°F														
37.15°C/99.1°F														
37.10°C/99.0°F														
37.05°C/98.9°F														
37.00°C/98.8°F														
36.95°C/98.7°F														
36.90°C/98.6°F														
36.85°C/98.5°F														
36.80°C/98.4°F														
36.75°C/98.3°F														
36.70°C/98.2°F														
36.65°C/98.1°F														
36.60°C/98.0°F														
36.55°C/97.9°F														
36.50°C/97.8°F														
36.45°C/97.7°F														
36.40°C/97.6°F														
36.35°C/97.5°F														
36.30°C/97.4°F														
36.25°C/97.3°F														
36.20°C/97.2°F														
36.15°C/97.1°F														
36.10°C/97.0°F														
36.05°C/96.9°F														
36.00°C/96.8°F														
35.95°C/96.7°F														
35.90°C/96.6°F														

Cervical fluid														
Cervical position														
Cervical texture														
Sex														
Ovulation test														
Pregnancy test														
Period														
Day of cycle														

CERVICAL FLUID: **S** – Sticky   **C** – Creamy   **W** – Watery   **E** – Egg white

CERVICAL POSITION: **L** – Low   **M** – Medium   **H** – High

CERVICAL TEXTURE: **S** – Soft   **M** – Medium   **F** – Firm

15	16	17	18	19	20	21	22	23	24	25	26	27	28	29	30	31

Symptoms & treatments

Month:

SYMPTOM:

	1	2	3	4	5	6	7	8	9	10	11	12	13	14	15	16	17	18	19	20	21	22	23	24	25	26	27	28	29	30	31
☺																															
☺																															
☺																															
☹																															
☹																															

SYMPTOM:

	1	2	3	4	5	6	7	8	9	10	11	12	13	14	15	16	17	18	19	20	21	22	23	24	25	26	27	28	29	30	31
☺																															
☺																															
☺																															
☹																															
☹																															

SYMPTOM:

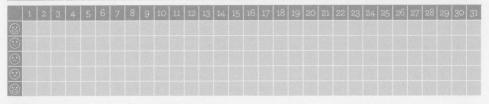

	1	2	3	4	5	6	7	8	9	10	11	12	13	14	15	16	17	18	19	20	21	22	23	24	25	26	27	28	29	30	31
☺																															
☺																															
☺																															
☹																															
☹																															

SYMPTOM:

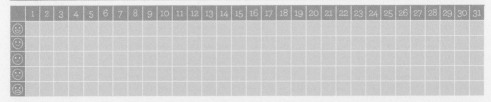

	1	2	3	4	5	6	7	8	9	10	11	12	13	14	15	16	17	18	19	20	21	22	23	24	25	26	27	28	29	30	31
☺																															
☺																															
☺																															
☹																															
☹																															

SYMPTOM:

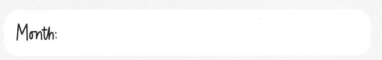

	1	2	3	4	5	6	7	8	9	10	11	12	13	14	15	16	17	18	19	20	21	22	23	24	25	26	27	28	29	30	31
☺																															
☺																															
☺																															
☹																															
☹																															

SYMPTOM: _____

	1	2	3	4	5	6	7	8	9	10	11	12	13	14	15	16	17	18	19	20	21	22	23	24	25	26	27	28	29	30	31
😀																															
🙂																															
😐																															
🙁																															
☹️																															

SYMPTOM: _____

	1	2	3	4	5	6	7	8	9	10	11	12	13	14	15	16	17	18	19	20	21	22	23	24	25	26	27	28	29	30	31
😀																															
🙂																															
😐																															
🙁																															
☹️																															

SYMPTOM: _____

	1	2	3	4	5	6	7	8	9	10	11	12	13	14	15	16	17	18	19	20	21	22	23	24	25	26	27	28	29	30	31
😀																															
🙂																															
😐																															
🙁																															
☹️																															

SYMPTOM: _____

	1	2	3	4	5	6	7	8	9	10	11	12	13	14	15	16	17	18	19	20	21	22	23	24	25	26	27	28	29	30	31
😀																															
🙂																															
😐																															
🙁																															
☹️																															

TREATMENT STARTED: **A** _____

B _____ C _____

D _____ E _____

F _____ G _____

	1	2	3	4	5	6	7	8	9	10	11	12	13	14	15	16	17	18	19	20	21	22	23	24	25	26	27	28	29	30	31
A																															
B																															
C																															
D																															
E																															
F																															
G																															

Habits

Month:

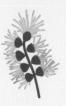

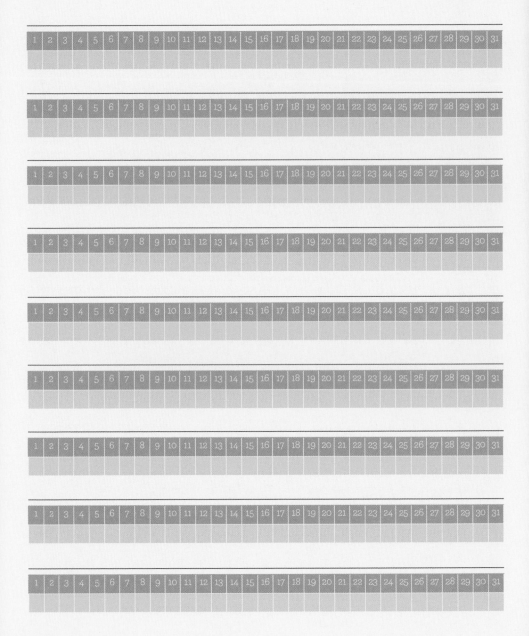

| 1 | 2 | 3 | 4 | 5 | 6 | 7 | 8 | 9 | 10 | 11 | 12 | 13 | 14 | 15 | 16 | 17 | 18 | 19 | 20 | 21 | 22 | 23 | 24 | 25 | 26 | 27 | 28 | 29 | 30 | 31 |

| 1 | 2 | 3 | 4 | 5 | 6 | 7 | 8 | 9 | 10 | 11 | 12 | 13 | 14 | 15 | 16 | 17 | 18 | 19 | 20 | 21 | 22 | 23 | 24 | 25 | 26 | 27 | 28 | 29 | 30 | 31 |

| 1 | 2 | 3 | 4 | 5 | 6 | 7 | 8 | 9 | 10 | 11 | 12 | 13 | 14 | 15 | 16 | 17 | 18 | 19 | 20 | 21 | 22 | 23 | 24 | 25 | 26 | 27 | 28 | 29 | 30 | 31 |

| 1 | 2 | 3 | 4 | 5 | 6 | 7 | 8 | 9 | 10 | 11 | 12 | 13 | 14 | 15 | 16 | 17 | 18 | 19 | 20 | 21 | 22 | 23 | 24 | 25 | 26 | 27 | 28 | 29 | 30 | 31 |

| 1 | 2 | 3 | 4 | 5 | 6 | 7 | 8 | 9 | 10 | 11 | 12 | 13 | 14 | 15 | 16 | 17 | 18 | 19 | 20 | 21 | 22 | 23 | 24 | 25 | 26 | 27 | 28 | 29 | 30 | 31 |

| 1 | 2 | 3 | 4 | 5 | 6 | 7 | 8 | 9 | 10 | 11 | 12 | 13 | 14 | 15 | 16 | 17 | 18 | 19 | 20 | 21 | 22 | 23 | 24 | 25 | 26 | 27 | 28 | 29 | 30 | 31 |

| 1 | 2 | 3 | 4 | 5 | 6 | 7 | 8 | 9 | 10 | 11 | 12 | 13 | 14 | 15 | 16 | 17 | 18 | 19 | 20 | 21 | 22 | 23 | 24 | 25 | 26 | 27 | 28 | 29 | 30 | 31 |

| 1 | 2 | 3 | 4 | 5 | 6 | 7 | 8 | 9 | 10 | 11 | 12 | 13 | 14 | 15 | 16 | 17 | 18 | 19 | 20 | 21 | 22 | 23 | 24 | 25 | 26 | 27 | 28 | 29 | 30 | 31 |

Weight

Month:

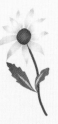

	1	2	3	4	5	6	7	8	9	10	11	12	13	14	15	16	17	18	19	20	21	22	23	24	25	26	27	28	29	30	31
W E I G H T																															

Cycle tracking

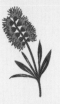

Month:

TEMPERATURE	1	2	3	4	5	6	7	8	9	10	11	12	13	14
37.30°C/99.4°F														
37.25°C/99.3°F														
37.20°C/99.2°F														
37.15°C/99.1°F														
37.10°C/99.0°F														
37.05°C/98.9°F														
37.00°C/98.8°F														
36.95°C/98.7°F														
36.90°C/98.6°F														
36.85°C/98.5°F														
36.80°C/98.4°F														
36.75°C/98.3°F														
36.70°C/98.2°F														
36.65°C/98.1°F														
36.60°C/98.0°F														
36.55°C/97.9°F														
36.50°C/97.8°F														
36.45°C/97.7°F														
36.40°C/97.6°F														
36.35°C/97.5°F														
36.30°C/97.4°F														
36.25°C/97.3°F														
36.20°C/97.2°F														
36.15°C/97.1°F														
36.10°C/97.0°F														
36.05°C/96.9°F														
36.00°C/96.8°F														
35.95°C/96.7°F														
35.90°C/96.6°F														

Cervical fluid														
Cervical position														
Cervical texture														
Sex														
Ovulation test														
Pregnancy test														
Period														
Day of cycle														

CERVICAL FLUID: **S** – Sticky   **C** – Creamy   **W** – Watery   **E** – Egg white

CERVICAL POSITION: **L** – Low   **M** – Medium   **H** – High

CERVICAL TEXTURE: **S** – Soft   **M** – Medium   **F** – Firm

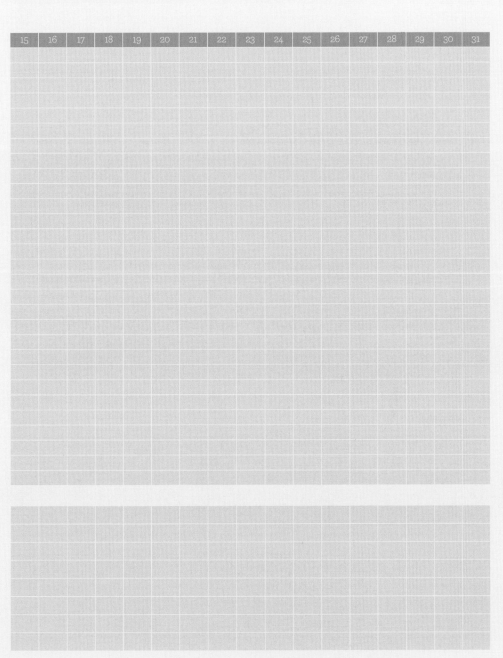

Symptoms & treatments

Month:

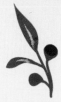

SYMPTOM:

	1	2	3	4	5	6	7	8	9	10	11	12	13	14	15	16	17	18	19	20	21	22	23	24	25	26	27	28	29	30	31
😄																															
🙂																															
😐																															
🙁																															
😞																															

SYMPTOM:

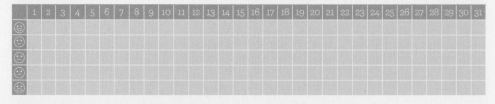

SYMPTOM:

	1	2	3	4	5	6	7	8	9	10	11	12	13	14	15	16	17	18	19	20	21	22	23	24	25	26	27	28	29	30	31
😄																															
🙂																															
😐																															
🙁																															
😞																															

SYMPTOM:

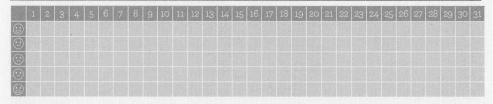

SYMPTOM:

	1	2	3	4	5	6	7	8	9	10	11	12	13	14	15	16	17	18	19	20	21	22	23	24	25	26	27	28	29	30	31
😄																															
🙂																															
😐																															
🙁																															
😞																															

SYMPTOM:

	1	2	3	4	5	6	7	8	9	10	11	12	13	14	15	16	17	18	19	20	21	22	23	24	25	26	27	28	29	30	31
😀																															
🙂																															
😐																															
🙁																															
😣																															

SYMPTOM:

	1	2	3	4	5	6	7	8	9	10	11	12	13	14	15	16	17	18	19	20	21	22	23	24	25	26	27	28	29	30	31
😀																															
🙂																															
😐																															
🙁																															
😣																															

SYMPTOM:

	1	2	3	4	5	6	7	8	9	10	11	12	13	14	15	16	17	18	19	20	21	22	23	24	25	26	27	28	29	30	31
😀																															
🙂																															
😐																															
🙁																															
😣																															

SYMPTOM:

	1	2	3	4	5	6	7	8	9	10	11	12	13	14	15	16	17	18	19	20	21	22	23	24	25	26	27	28	29	30	31
😀																															
🙂																															
😐																															
🙁																															
😣																															

TREATMENT STARTED: **A**

B _____ C _____

D _____ E _____

F _____ G _____

	1	2	3	4	5	6	7	8	9	10	11	12	13	14	15	16	17	18	19	20	21	22	23	24	25	26	27	28	29	30	31
A																															
B																															
C																															
D																															
E																															
F																															
G																															

Habits

Month:

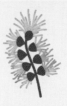

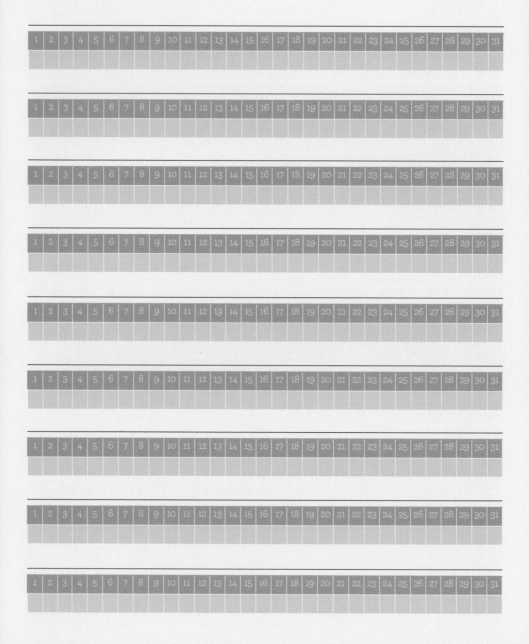

1	2	3	4	5	6	7	8	9	10	11	12	13	14	15	16	17	18	19	20	21	22	23	24	25	26	27	28	29	30	31

Weight

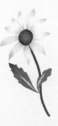

Month:

WEIGHT		1	2	3	4	5	6	7	8	9	10	11	12	13	14	15	16	17	18	19	20	21	22	23	24	25	26	27	28	29	30	31

Cycle tracking

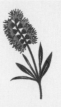

Month:

TEMPERATURE	1	2	3	4	5	6	7	8	9	10	11	12	13	14
37.30°C/99.4°F														
37.25°C/99.3°F														
37.20°C/99.2°F														
37.15°C/99.1°F														
37.10°C/99.0°F														
37.05°C/98.9°F														
37.00°C/98.8°F														
36.95°C/98.7°F														
36.90°C/98.6°F														
36.85°C/98.5°F														
36.80°C/98.4°F														
36.75°C/98.3°F														
36.70°C/98.2°F														
36.65°C/98.1°F														
36.60°C/98.0°F														
36.55°C/97.9°F														
36.50°C/97.8°F														
36.45°C/97.7°F														
36.40°C/97.6°F														
36.35°C/97.5°F														
36.30°C/97.4°F														
36.25°C/97.3°F														
36.20°C/97.2°F														
36.15°C/97.1°F														
36.10°C/97.0°F														
36.05°C/96.9°F														
36.00°C/96.8°F														
35.95°C/96.7°F														
35.90°C/96.6°F														

Cervical fluid														
Cervical position														
Cervical texture														
Sex														
Ovulation test														
Pregnancy test														
Period														
Day of cycle														

CERVICAL FLUID: **S** – Sticky   **C** – Creamy   **W** – Watery   **E** – Egg white

CERVICAL POSITION: **L** – Low   **M** – Medium   **H** – High

CERVICAL TEXTURE: **S** – Soft   **M** – Medium   **F** – Firm

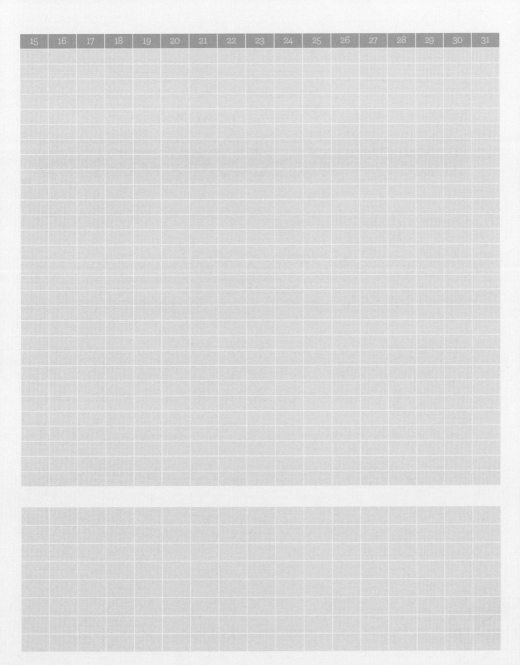

15	16	17	18	19	20	21	22	23	24	25	26	27	28	29	30	31

TEST RESULTS

It is important to understand what is happening in your body and keep up to date with its changes. A general blood test once or twice per year can help you achieve this understanding.

Our recommendation is to do your research and request the tests you want done. Try to establish a working relationship with your doctor so you can improve your health together. If you don't feel like you are a team working together, we encourage you to seek a new doctor until you find one who fits.

TEST	RESULT 1	RESULT 2

TEST	RESULT 1	RESULT 2

WHAT DO YOUR CYCLE PHASES FEEL LIKE??

Throughout the charts section you will find your cycle tracking charts, which you can use to record the factual details of your cycle like cervical fluid and body temp.

This chart isn't that.

This chart is here for you to make notes throughout the year about what your experience of each cycle phase feels like. If you haven't already, read about the cycle phases in Chapter 3 of the journal.

For example, you might notice that in your luteal phase, you like to watch more TV or you like to write more. Or in your ovulatory phase, you might find that you feel super charismatic at work.

Consider what your energy levels are like, how introverted you feel, if studying comes easily, how confident you feel, what your temperament is like, how much you enjoy exercise, and how focused you are at work or on projects.

Whatever you notice, it's all interesting and valid.

If you continue to add your observations to this chart throughout the year, by the end of the year (or probably sooner) you might have a really detailed idea of what each cycle phase is like for you. And moving forward, you will be able to use that info when making plans – everything from throwing parties to launching products to locking in first dates.

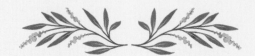

MENSTRUAL PHASE
Starts day 1 of your cycle until
when your period ends

FOLLICULAR PHASE
Starts day 1 of your cycle
until you ovulate

OVULATORY PHASE
The few days leading up to
and including ovulation

LUTEAL PHASE
Starts the day after ovulation and
ends when you get your period

LET'S REFLECT

I t's been a year and if you're here reading this, it's probably been a year where you have learnt a lot about health and a lot about yourself! It's time to reflect. So make a cuppa or pour a glass and delve into the year that was ...

Your cycle

Did you find that your cycle was a typical length?

_____

_____

What was the average length of your cycle?

_____

_____

Did you find that your period was typical?

_____

_____

Did you suffer from PMS?

_____

_____

Did you make any changes to improve your cycle?

_____

_____

How do you feel about your cycle – do you have a better understanding of it? Do you feel more connected to it?

_____

_____

Is there anything you want to work on to improve your cycle health?

_____

_____

Your lifestyle

Did you find any self-care practices that you loved? What were they?

_____

_____

_____

Have you made time to include self-care regularly?

_____

_____

_____

Have you found a way of eating that suits you and feels good?

_____

_____

_____

How has your sleep been?

_____

_____

_____

Are you happy with how much body movement you've been including in your life?

_____

_____

Do you feel like you've made a positive lifestyle shift this year?

_____

_____

Is there anything you want to work on to improve your lifestyle?

_____

_____

_____

Your health care

Have you found a healthcare professional who you love?

_____

_____

_____

_____

_____

Have you started any treatments that have worked really well for you?

_____

_____

_____

_____

_____

Are there any modalities you would like to explore that you haven't already?

_____

_____

_____

_____

_____

Do you feel like you're on a great treatment path or would you want to explore something new?

_____

_____

_____

_____

_____

Your journey

Do you feel like you have a better understanding of your body?

_____

_____

_____

Does your health feel in a better or worse place than it was at the beginning of the year?

_____

_____

_____

Do you feel like the relationship with your body has improved?

_____

_____

How is your mental health? Do you feel like you've got support and an effective management plan for your mental health if you need it?

_____

_____

_____

How knowledgeable do you feel about health?

_____

_____

Have you shared anything you've learnt?

_____

_____

How did you go with your intentions this year? Are there some you can tick off? Others you would like to continue working on?

_____

_____

You did it! Twelve months of knowledge building and dedicated self-love, self-care and self-reflection. We hope you have a deeper connection with your body and feel filled with wisdom about how to protect and improve your health. If you need somewhere to talk about all things health – join us in the My Wellness Journal Book Club – facebook.com/groups/mywellnessjournalbookclub – we hope to see you there!

Mel and Steph xo

A Rockpool book
PO Box 252
Summer Hill
NSW 2130
Australia

rockpoolpublishing.com
Follow us! f ⃝ rockpoolpublishing
Tag your images with #rockpoolpublishing

ISBN: 9781922579430

Published in 2023 by Rockpool Publishing
Copyright text © Melissa Christie 2023
Copyright illustrations © Stephanie Crane 2023
Copyright design © Rockpool Publishing 2023

MEDICAL DISCLAIMER The information provided in this book is designed to provide helpful information on the subjects discussed. This book is not meant to be used, nor should it be used, to diagnose or treat any medical condition. For diagnosis or treatment of any medical problem, consult your own healthcare practitioner. The author is not responsible for any health needs that may require medical supervision and is not liable for any damages or negative consequences from any treatment, action, application or preparation, to any person reading or following the information in this book.

Special thanks to our brilliant advisory team of health practitioners who read over the manuscript for this journal to ensure it was medically accurate:

Myra Lewin – @hale_pule
Jessica Maguire – @repairing_the_nervous_system
Kimberley Peters – @_kimberleypeters
Rachel Vong – @drvongnd
Brie Wieselman – @briewieselman

Design by Sara Lindberg, Rockpool Publishing

Printed and bound in China
10 9 8 7 6 5 4 3 2 1

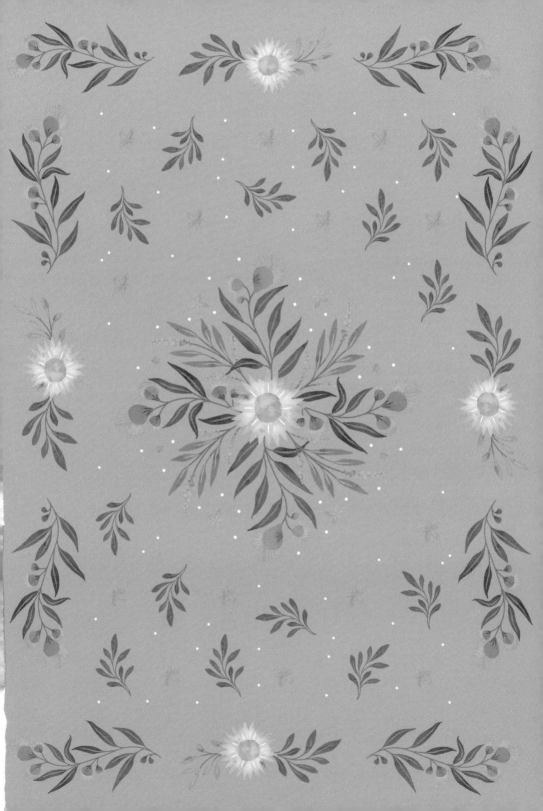

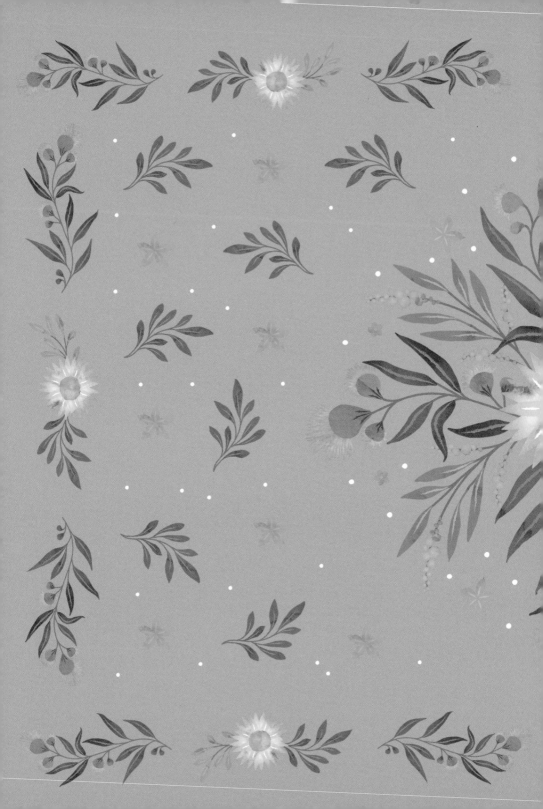